Fighting Lupus Battles

Living
   Hoping
      Searching
         Climbing
            Researching
               for the Cure

Kayrene Mimms

Hilton Publishing Company
5261-A Fountain Drive
Crown Point, IN 46307
219-922-4868
www.hiltonpub.com

Copyright © 2019 by Kayrene Mimms
ISBN (print) 978-0-9777779-9-0
ISBN (ebook) 978-0-9773160-0-7

Notice: The information in this book is true and complete to the best of the author's and publisher's knowledge. This book is intended only as an information reference and should not replace, countermand, or conflict with the advice given to readers by their physicians. The author and publisher disclaim all liability in connection with the specific personal use of any and all information provided in this book.

All rights reserved. No part of this book may be reproduced or transmitted in any form or by any means, electronic or mechanical, including photocopy, recording, or any information storage or retrieval systems, including digital systems, without written permission from the publisher, except by a reviewer who may quote brief passages from the book in a review.

Angela Vennemann, Senior Editor and Design
Judine O'Shea, Publisher
Megan Lippert, Executive Vice President, Hilton Publishing Division

Cover concept created by John M. Davis and Michal Davis
LSI Body Chart created by Eric DesBiens and provided by the Lupus Society of Illinois (LSI)
Additional editing by Helena Fields
Photographs and other images provided by Cecil Mimms, Jr.; Dana Mimms, Sr.; author; and contributing writers
Collages designed by Cecil Mimms, Jr.

Library of Congress Cataloging-in-Publication Data

Names: Mimms, Kayrene, compiler.
Title: Fighting lupus battles : living, hoping, searching, climbing, researching for the cure / Kayrene Mimms.
Description: Crown Point, IN : Hilton Publishing Company, [2019] | Originally published: 2015. | Includes bibliographical references.
Identifiers: LCCN 2019017571 (print) | LCCN 2019017980 (ebook) | ISBN 9780977316007 (ebook) | ISBN 9780977777990
Subjects: LCSH: Systemic lupus erythematosus—Personal narratives.
Classification: LCC RC924.5.L85 (ebook) | LCC RC924.5.L85 M56 2019 (print) | DDC 616.7/72—dc23
LC record available at https://lccn.loc.gov/2019017571

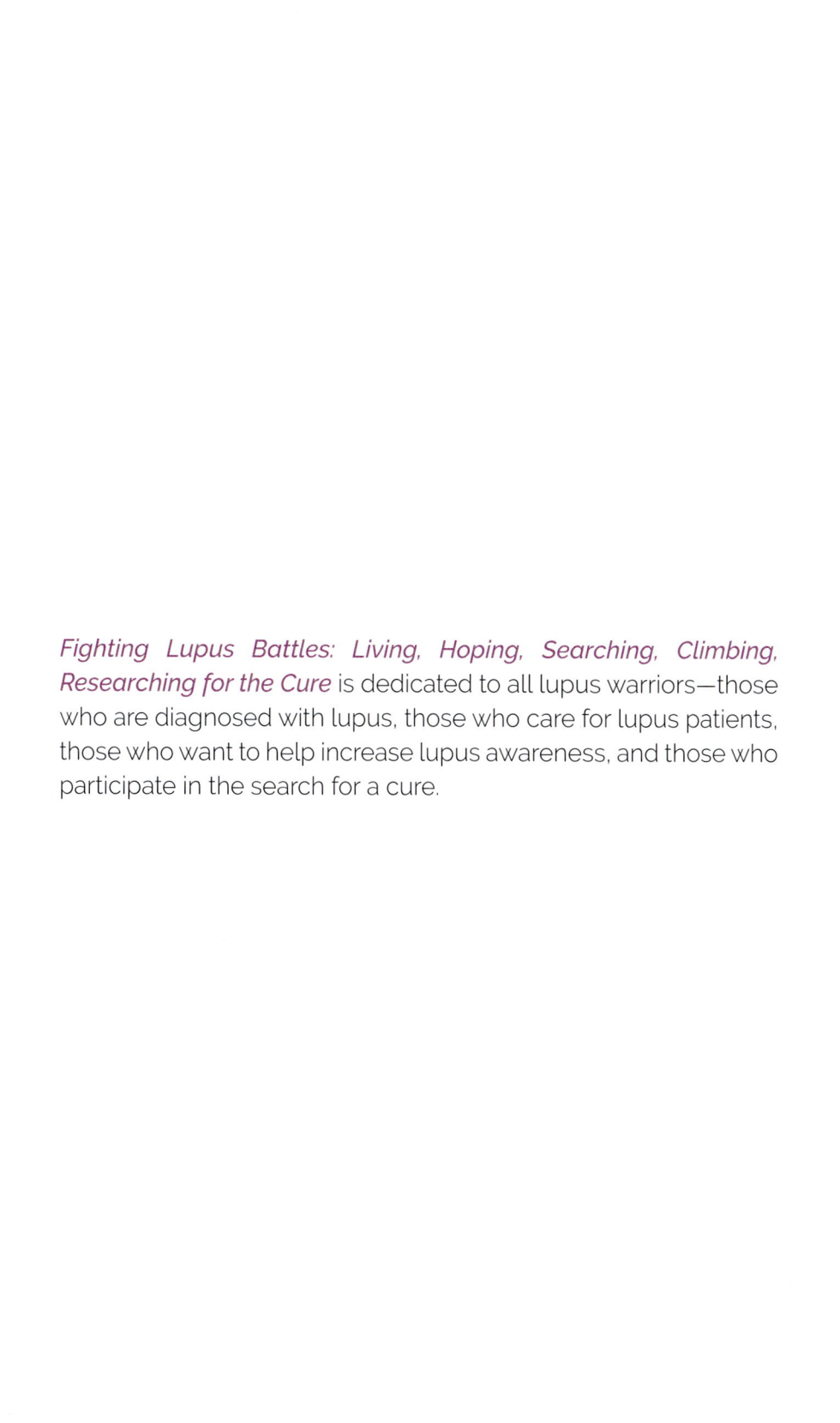

Fighting Lupus Battles: Living, Hoping, Searching, Climbing, Researching for the Cure is dedicated to all lupus warriors—those who are diagnosed with lupus, those who care for lupus patients, those who want to help increase lupus awareness, and those who participate in the search for a cure.

Contents

Acknowledgments — ix
Author's Disclaimer — xii
Introduction — xiii

Part I—Living With Lupus

About Lupus — 3
    Robert S. Katz, MD

Section 1—*Fighting Lupus Battles: Hope For A Cure* Updates

Still Learning To Live Well With Lupus — 8
    Kayrene Mimms

A History With God — 12
    Robinzina "Zina" Bryant

The Other Side Of Fear: My Life Despite Lupus — 15
    Ashley Chappell-Rice

Fortunate And Grateful — 22
    Tari Ambler

Just Like That: Another Chance At Life — 23
    Ivy M. Douglas

Fighting And Hoping For The Best — 29
    Helena Fields

Lupus Lessons — 33
    Patricia L. Sanders

Vision: Living A Life Without Lupus — 35
    Sarah Spadoni, CVT

In Remission: My Life With Lupus, Part II — 41
    Kanefus R. Walker

Section 2—Journeys Of More Lupus Warriors

Gentle Hugs & Hope — 48
"BB"

The Newest Addition To The Branch Family — 55
Duwana Branch

Lupus Survivor And Advocate: I'm Blessed — 61
Patricia A. Brumley

Name That Disease: What Is Lupus? — 64
Bettie Carter

Lupus: My Beginnings, No End! — 72
Donna L. Emery

Finding Understanding: Hoping For A Cure — 75
Chris Fragassi

Lupus Testimony — 79
Jasmine Henderson

My Lupus Story — 85
Gloria Morris

Unwavering Faith And Courage — 88
Sherry Y. Sims

Part II—Finding Answers Through Research

What Clinical Research Means To You — 103
Kenneth Getz and Ellyn Getz

Interview With Shanelle Gabriel — 112
Ellyn Getz

African-American Participation In Lupus Clinical Research: Why It Matters — 115
Rodlescia S. Sneed, PhD, MPH

My Lupus Research Experiences — 119
Kayrene Mimms

Development Of Patient Reported Outcomes Tools — 135
Meenakshi Jolly, MD

Bench-to-Bedside Model — 138
Kichul Ko, MD

The Activity In Lupus To Energize And Renew (ALTER) Study — 141
Rosalind Ramsey-Goldman, MD, DrPH

Lupus Research Alliance Delivering Research Breakthroughs To Transform Lupus Treatment — 145
Teodora P. Staeva, PhD

The Lupus Research Community — 149
Scott Hadly, 23Andme, Inc.

Research.forME™ Lupus Registry — 151
The Lupus Foundation Of America

Part III—Summary

Summary — 155

References/Resources — 159

Acknowledgments

My sincere appreciation goes out to all who helped in bringing this project to completion. Fellow lupus warriors have shared details about some of their trials and triumphs while fighting lupus battles. I commend all who are brave and courageous enough to describe events that they experience while dealing with lupus. The lupus warriors who shared their stories for this book are:

Ashley Chappell-Rice
Bettie Carter
Chris Fragassi
Donna L. Emery
Duwana Branch
Gloria Morris
Helena Fields
Ivy M. Douglas
Jasmine Henderson
Kanefus R. Walker
Patricia A. Brumley
Patricia L. Sanders
Robbin Zaffini
Robinzina "Zina" Bryant
Sarah Spadoni, C.V.T.
Shanelle Gabriel
Sherry Y. Sims
Tari Ambler

I sincerely appreciate my doctor, Dr. Rosalind Ramsey-Goldman, for providing written commentary for each contributor's story.

I am very grateful to the coordinators, directors, doctors, founders, managers, principal investigators, and professors of lupus research clinics, companies, and organizations. All took time out of their very busy schedules to give brief descriptions of some of their contributions to lupus care and research. They include:

Fighting Lupus Battles

Ellyn Getz, senior manager, Development & Community Engagement, Center for Information and Study on Clinical Research Participation (CISCRP)

Kenneth Getz, associate professor, Tufts University; founder, Center for Information and Study on Clinical Research Participation (CISCRP)

Scott Hadly, 23andMe, Inc.

Meenakshi Jolly, MD, director, Rush Lupus Clinic at Rush University Medical Center

Robert S. Katz, MD, professor of medicine at Northwestern University's Feinberg School of Medicine and Rush Medical School

Kichul Ko, MD, assistant professor of medicine at The University of Chicago

The Lupus Foundation of America

Rosalind Ramsey-Goldman, MD, DrPH, Solovy Arthritis Research Society professor of medicine, Northwestern University, Feinberg School of Medicine

Rodlescia S. Sneed, PhD, MPH, assistant professor, Michigan State University

Teodora P. Staeva, PhD, research director, Lupus Research Alliance.

I express special thanks to attorney David C. Hilliard of Pattishall, McAuliffe, Newbury, Hilliard & Geraldson LLP for providing pro bono legal advice.

Artist John M. Davis created the concept for the book cover for which his wife, Michal Davis, modeled. Thank you very much, John and Michal.

Acknowledgments

I would also like to express words of gratitude to my supporters who provided encouragement, inspiration, editing, review, and recommendations. They include:

>Charles Brummell, CEO, Lupus Society of Illinois (LSI)
>Helena Fields
>Virginia A. Mitamura
>Lewis Nixon
>Beverly Rogers
>Janice Stewart
>Dr. Deborah Terrell.

I sincerely thank Dr. Hilton M. Hudson, II, president and CEO of Hilton Publishing Company (HPC), for accepting my proposal. Also thanks to Megan Lippert, Judine O'Shea, and Angela Vennemann, who provided assistance in the publishing process. I am most grateful to God and my husband, Cecil. God planted the seed for this book, and Cecil provided support and encouragement that helped it become a fully-grown plant. To God be the Glory.

Author's Disclaimer

The purpose of this book, *Fighting Lupus Battles: Living, Hoping, Searching, Climbing, Researching for the Cure*, is to increase lupus awareness and encourage more participation in lupus research. I am not a medical professional, and I do not claim to be a lupus expert in any way. Rather, I am an individual who, after being diagnosed with lupus, wants to share my story, the stories of other lupus patients, and information about lupus research with the world.

The contributors to this book have guaranteed that their stories represent factual accounts of their experiences. We provide this information to help shed light on the complexity of this disease and possible ways to find a cure, not to offer any professional advice or services.

The scientific information found in this book about lupus was taken from publications provided by the American College of Rheumatology (ACR), Center for Information and Study on Clinical Research Participation (CISCRP), Centers for Disease Control and Prevention (CDC), the Lupus Foundation of America, Inc. (LFA), the Lupus Research Alliance (LRA), the Lupus Society of Illinois (LSI), the National Cancer Institute (NCI), the National Institute of Arthritis and Musculoskeletal and Skin Diseases (NIAMS), and the National Institutes of Health (NIH).

The author and other participants shall not be held liable or responsible to any person or entity for loss or damage caused or alleged to be caused directly or indirectly by the information contained in this book. If you or someone you know has any of the symptoms that are discussed in this book, we recommend that you seek professional medical advice as soon as possible.

Introduction

Why a second book about lupus?

In my first book, *Fighting Lupus Battles: Hope for a Cure*, patients, relatives, and doctors wrote about their experiences with lupus. As I attended lupus awareness events, many who read the first book wanted to know more about the contributors' lives today. I was approached with questions like, "How are they doing? Why don't you ask them to write updates?" All I could say was, "As far as I know, all of us are still alive." Then other lupus patients expressed interest in sharing their stories as well. Those conversations gave birth to this sequel. One main objective is for readers to hear from those who have to deal with lupus on a daily basis.

Other conversations made it apparent to me that lupus awareness still has a long way to go. There's still a lot of misinformation. There are still many unanswered questions surrounding lupus. I concluded that more research could be a powerful avenue for solving the mysteries. I determined that additional objectives would be for readers to:

- gain insight into the need for and importance of lupus research
- have a better understanding of the lupus research process
- become aware of the need for more volunteers in lupus research
- feel more comfortable volunteering to participate in lupus research.

Fighting Lupus Battles

I consider "the world" as being my intended audience, especially those affected by lupus, those who may have lupus symptoms, those who want to help increase lupus awareness, and those who want to join the search for a cure. Writing this book has been very difficult, and I almost gave up several times. At first, I was excited and highly motivated as I received stories from fellow lupus warriors. I was moving forward with the first section of the book. However, the task of completing the research section was daunting. I am not a medical professional. In fact, I have no medical training. So I felt very incompetent as I tried to develop convincing arguments that would encourage participation in lupus research. I've been involved in several nonintervention or observational studies, which I write about later in this book, but I knew very little about trials or interventional studies. So I reached out to principal investigators who are involved in lupus research as well as companies and organizations that promote, support, and sponsor lupus research. Several responded positively and wrote brief summaries about some of their involvement in lupus research. Their contributions are extremely important in helping readers understand the process and benefits of lupus research.

Beverly Rogers, certified institutional review board (IRB) member, sat with me and provided materials so I could get a better understanding of the IRB process. Beverly explained the ins and outs of clinical research studies to me, including the rights of study participants, questions participants should ask the study authors, and safety mechanisms that are in place to protect study participants. She also encouraged me along the way, and her advice propelled me forward in completing this project.

Meeting Ellyn Getz at a CISCRP event was one of the best things that could have happened for me. Not only did she provide a copy of her father's book, *The Gift of Participation* by Kenneth Getz, but she also wrote a critical piece in this book's research section, introduced me to lupus research participants, and provided general

Introduction

encouragement. Thank you, Ellyn. Finally, a book like this would not be possible without the stories that were shared by our courageous writers. Thank you very much.

I pray this book will help readers to learn more about lupus and to be encouraged to join us in the struggle to develop a world without lupus. Let's search for the cure.

Part I
Living With Lupus

What is lupus?

Living with a chronic (long-lasting) and often unpredictable disease like lupus can be very stressful. The American College of Rheumatology says that "lupus flares vary from mild to serious. Most patients have times when the disease is active, followed by times when the disease is mostly quiet—referred to as a remission."[1]

Part I begins with Dr. Robert S. Katz's article, "About Lupus," in which he provides a description of the disease called lupus. Next are updates from lupus warriors who shared their stories in the first book, followed by reflections from more lupus warriors on their experiences. The purpose of Part I is to provide an opportunity for readers to get a realistic view of trials and triumphs for those who deal with lupus on a daily basis.

---

1 American College of Rheumatology, https://www.rheumatology.org/I-Am-A/Patient-Caregiver/Diseases-Conditions/Lupus

About Lupus

Robert S. Katz, MD

Dr. Katz is a professor of medicine at Northwestern University's Feinberg School of Medicine and Rush Medical College.

SYSTEMIC LUPUS ERYTHEMATOSUS (SLE), commonly called lupus, is an immune system disorder that may affect many organs of the body, including the skin, joints, heart, lungs, kidneys, brain, and/or blood vessels. The immune system produces small antibodies that protect the body against viruses and foreign substances. However, in lupus patients, the antibodies appear to attack healthy cells and tissues, leading to inflammation and damage in the patient's organs.

The most common symptoms of lupus are fatigue, painful and swollen joints, morning stiffness, fever over 100°F for an extended period of time, and skin rashes, particularly on sun-exposed areas such as the face. Other symptoms may include chest pain with deep breathing (due to inflammation around the heart or lungs), unusual amounts of hair loss, and white or blue fingertips with exposure to cold (a condition known as Raynaud's disease). Symptoms may also include paleness from anemia, neurological problems like confusion and seizures, and ulcers in the mouth or nose for more than a few days at a time.

Self-diagnosis is discouraged because many people suspect they have the disease without having the necessary medical evidence. Other conditions, such as rheumatoid arthritis, fibromyalgia, and chronic fatigue syndrome, may share similar symptoms. Primary care physicians and rheumatologists collect the individual's

Fighting Lupus Battles

symptoms and medical history, conduct a physical examination, and order lab tests before making a lupus diagnosis. Once a diagnosis has been firmly established, patients are assessed for damage to major organs, including the central nervous system, kidneys, heart, or lungs. Other specialists such as nephrologists (for kidney involvement), dermatologists (for skin involvement), neurologists (for brain involvement), and hematologists (for blood abnormalities) may treat patients who have major organ problems. Treatment is tailored to the activity and severity of the disease. Many lupus patients have benign disease without major organ involvement and have a favorable course of treatment. Treatment given in the early stages of lupus may reduce the patient's chances of suffering permanent organ damage.

Some patients try dietary supplements and herbal medications on their own to help treat the disease, but these therapies have not been studied thoroughly in systemic lupus patients. No one knows what effect, if any, supplements may have.

Physicians, usually specialists such as rheumatologists, monitor the patient continually with laboratory tests that include complete blood counts, urinalysis, blood chemistry measurements, sedimentation rate measurements, antibody tests, and blood complement levels. It is important that physicians monitor the patient's symptoms regularly to determine the success of the treatment.

Patients are often treated with the antimalarial drug hydroxychloroquine (Plaquenil); nonsteroidal anti-inflammatory drugs (NSAIDs), such as naproxen (Aleve, Naprosyn) and ibuprofen (Advil, Motrin); or the NSAIDs known as COX-2 inhibitors (Celebrex). If a lupus patient is running a fever or has major organ involvement, the treating physician generally prescribes corticosteroids such as prednisone, sometimes at high doses initially that are then tapered to a small dosage or discontinued. The dosage depends on the type of organ involvement, the patient's symptoms, blood-test results, and any side effects caused by the steroid.

About Lupus

Drugs that suppress the immune system may be helpful in controlling the overactive but misdirected immune system in lupus patients. These drugs include azathioprine (Imuran), methotrexate, leflunomide (Arava), cyclophosphamide (Cytoxan), cyclosporine (Neoral), mycophenolate mofetil (CellCept), tacrolimus (Prograf) and rituximab (Rituxan). Belimumab (Benlysta), a B lymphocyte white blood cell inhibitor, is given intravenously once a month. Additional biologic response medications similar to Benlysta are currently being studied for lupus treatment.

Lupus occurs predominantly in young women. In fact, women are nine times more likely than men to be diagnosed with lupus. Additionally, lupus is much more common in women of childbearing age than in premenstrual or post-menopausal women. Animal studies have shown that there is a hormonal connection between the symptoms of lupus and the body's immune system.

Although studies have shown that lupus tends to run in families and has a genetic basis, the offspring of lupus patients are affected only about 5% of the time. However, family members of lupus patients often test positive for lupus antibodies, though they may not develop any symptoms of the disease.

African-American, Latina-American, Native-American, and Asian women have higher rates of lupus than Caucasian women, presumably due to a genetic susceptibility to the disease. While some of the genes associated with a susceptibility to lupus have been identified, scientists do not know the exact combinations of genes that make some individuals more likely to have the disease.

Lupus tends to occur in flare periods when the disease is more active. In between the flare-ups, patients may be completely without symptoms. No one knows for sure what triggers the flare periods. Occasionally, sunlight, medications, stress, or pregnancy are the precipitating factors, but often the specific trigger is not known.

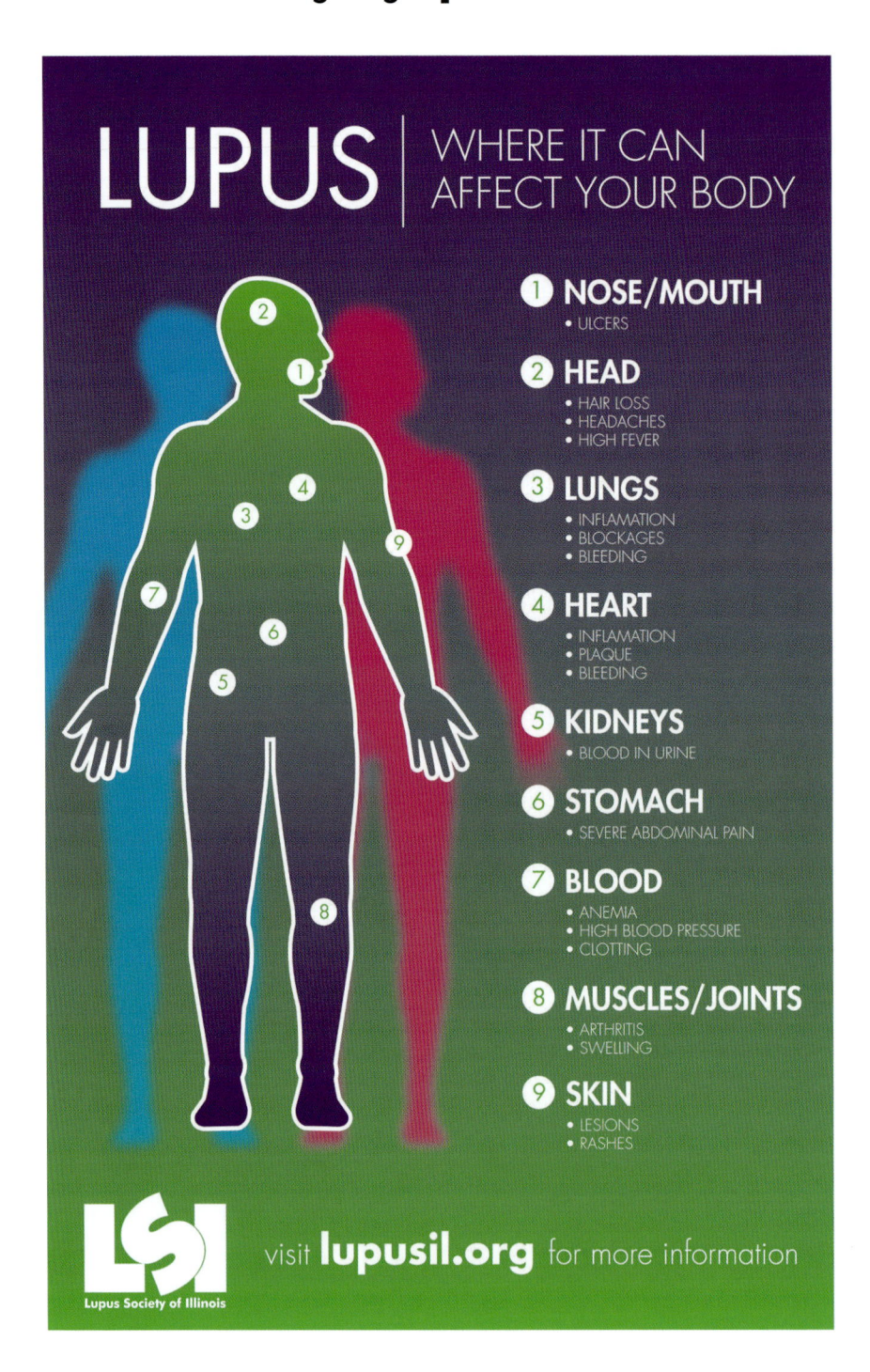

Fighting Lupus Battles

LUPUS | WHERE IT CAN AFFECT YOUR BODY

1. **NOSE/MOUTH**
   - ULCERS

2. **HEAD**
   - HAIR LOSS
   - HEADACHES
   - HIGH FEVER

3. **LUNGS**
   - INFLAMATION
   - BLOCKAGES
   - BLEEDING

4. **HEART**
   - INFLAMATION
   - PLAQUE
   - BLEEDING

5. **KIDNEYS**
   - BLOOD IN URINE

6. **STOMACH**
   - SEVERE ABDOMINAL PAIN

7. **BLOOD**
   - ANEMIA
   - HIGH BLOOD PRESSURE
   - CLOTTING

8. **MUSCLES/JOINTS**
   - ARTHRITIS
   - SWELLING

9. **SKIN**
   - LESIONS
   - RASHES

LSI — Lupus Society of Illinois

visit **lupusil.org** for more information

Section I
Fighting Lupus Battles: Hope For a Cure Updates

A SECTION OF OUR first book, *Fighting Lupus Battles: Hope for a Cure*, includes detailed accounts about personal trials and triumphs from several individuals who received a lupus diagnosis. Readers are given the opportunity to learn about the writers' responses to the initial diagnosis, get a glimpse of how close friends and family members were affected, review treatment plans that highlighted successes and failures, and gain insight into the unique ability of individuals to embrace their "new normal" for living and coping with lupus. While the war against this chronic disease continues, it is my hope that as you read this section, you will be encouraged to join us as we continue to search for a cure.

Still Learning to Live Well with Lupus

Kayrene Mimms

I SPENT SOME TIME debating whether to include this story in the book because it is so personal and is not directly related to lupus. However, I decided to use it as a great example to demonstrate how we are always questioning if a health issue is caused by lupus or not.

As I sit in this very small room at the lupus clinic and wait for Patti, my nurse practitioner (NP), I'm feeling a little sorry for her. All the doctors must be here today because Patti is assigned to the little room near the bone density testing area. Patti enters, and with her usual friendly attitude, she greets me. I tease her about the room, but it doesn't seem to bother her. I give her my notes that describe what's been happening with me since the last visit three months ago.

After reviewing my notes, she asks me, "When are you going to take care of that?"

She is referring to my feeling of incomplete elimination, discomfort in my lower right abdominal area, and intermittent incontinence. These are a few of the issues that I've included in my notes for several months. Honestly, I had been so focused on my basic lupus issues of managing seventeen meds throughout the day and night, proper application of skin moisturizer and sunscreen all over my body, staying on my exercise plan, maintaining a proper diet, attending lupus events and health fairs, keeping appointments with doctors, and just living day to day that I didn't want to go after another project. But Patti doesn't give up.

Still Learning to Live Well with Lupus

She goes on to say, "They can probably do something about that, and it may not involve surgery. Why not check it out? One of my coworkers was very pleased with our gastroenterologists.[1] At least talk with them about your condition, and see what they say."

I didn't want to hear Patti's lecture again, so I saw the GI specialist before my next visit with her. She was right. The GI specialist and his assistant made me feel very comfortable until they described the tests that they wanted me to take. The first test, called anorectal manometry, sounded OK. My GI and his assistant explained that the anorectal manometry would allow them to measure the pressures of my rectum and anal sphincters. They went on to say that the test would also measure how well I could feel different sensations of fullness in my rectum. Primarily, it would give them documentation of how the rectal sphincter muscles work, how strong the sphincter muscles are, and if they relax as they should when having a bowel movement. I was thinking, *OK, I've gotten through two natural childbirths, so maybe I can handle this.*

The description of the second test—defecating proctogram—blew me away. My understanding was that I would have to drink a mixture that would cause me to defecate. The kicker was that pictures would be taken during elimination. I thought, *NO WAY. Using the bathroom is a very private matter.*

Finally, I decided to schedule the first test—anorectal manometry. When I called to schedule, I was told that I would have to administer two Fleet enemas on the day of the test. *Wait a minute.*

I asked, "Who administers the enemas?"

The scheduler answered, "The patient does the enemas."

Then I asked, "Can someone administer the enemas at the hospital?"

She answered, "No. You have to do it at home."

---

1   Gastroenterologists are referred to as GI doctors. They focus on the digestive system and its disorders.

Fighting Lupus Battles

My response: "But I live about forty miles from the hospital and don't know how I might react to the enemas. Will I have a bowel movement right away? Will I be able to hold it? Should I wear an astronaut diaper?"

The assistants suggested that I do one enema the night before the test and the second one before leaving home to take the test. They assured me that I would be OK and not poop on myself. So I scheduled the test, and it went well. It was determined that I had pelvic floor weakness and didn't need to do the defecating proctogram. Thank God. Instead, the GI specialist recommended pelvic floor physical therapy (PFPT) to strengthen my pelvic floor muscles. I'd never heard of that before and was skeptical. But they convinced me that though it takes time and persistence, PFPT is usually 90 percent effective.

I started PFPT at a women's health clinic. It mainly involved stretching, deep-breathing exercises, abdominal and lower back massages, contractions, light endurance training on a stationary bike, heat, a couple of rectal exams to measure muscle strength, and dietary recommendations of more fiber and water. I also discovered that my digestive system didn't do very well with four cups of coffee each morning and several squares of Ghirardelli chocolate in the afternoon. The PFPT went very well and was very successful. Though the discomfort in my lower right abdominal area still happens occasionally, the feeling of incomplete elimination and the intermittent incontinence seldom occur.

Later I asked the GI doctor if my digestive problems could be related to lupus. He emailed this note to me: "I'm glad you are feeling better. As you know, lupus is a disease with a very broad range of symptoms. But to my knowledge there is no relationship between the two. Keep going with the exercises on your own time to make sure things don't return to the way they were before."

My husband, Cecil, has branded me as his "come a long way, baby." I suffered from various lupus-like symptoms at different

Still Learning to Live Well with Lupus

times throughout my life. Finally at age fifty-nine, I received a definite diagnosis and almost died about two weeks later. I tell about my struggles, fears, losses, and victories in my first book, *Fighting Lupus Battles: Hope for a Cure*. The book includes more than 20 true stories about real people who are living with the effects of this mysterious and unpredictable disease called lupus. With medical commentary from two of my doctors, as well as general educational information about the disease, *Fighting Lupus Battles: Hope for a Cure* was written to raise awareness, broaden knowledge, encourage understanding and compassion, improve provider/patient communication and relationships, and promote research.

Thank God that today my condition is stable. I try to express gratitude for every day that I am still alive and am able to take care of myself. I awake each day being thankful to God that even though I have painful and sore joints and find it difficult to walk sometimes; even though my voice is raspy and I am not able to sing like I used to; even though I still have a mild productive cough; even though I fatigue easily; even though I forget or may not fully understand things at times; even though I second-guess most things I do; even though I have to take lots of medications, I AM STILL ALIVE and learning to live with lupus in a positive and productive way. I try to do what I can to be as healthy as possible, and I leave the rest to God.

Commentary by Dr. Rosalind Ramsey-Goldman

Developing a partnership with your healthcare provider is a key element in empowering yourself to deal with a chronic illness. Keeping a list of questions and concerns, even if the problem is not lupus-related, is helpful so you are ready to review them at the time of your visit.

A History with God

Robinzina "Zina" Bryant

MY KIDNEY TRANSPLANT from seven years ago is doing great, but 33 days ago, I received a new diagnosis. I heard the doctor say, "You have cancer." Those were the last words I ever expected to hear, but cancer is my new reality. When I initially agreed to be a part of the follow-up to the first *Fighting Lupus Battles* book, I had some ideas of what sorts of things I would write about. My law practice, which I began while still on dialysis, is flourishing. I initially thought I'd write about that. My grandson, whose birth in the midst of the worst of my illness gave me a reason, hope, and will to live, just turned 10 years old and is still the apple of my eye. I initially thought I would write about him. My daughter, who was often times a challenge to raise because she was strong-willed and rebellious, is now independent—still strong-willed but now counted among my best friends. I initially thought I would write about her. I have experienced a kidney transplant with no rejection issues over the last seven years. I initially thought I would write about that. I have been dating a great guy and just might reach that one yet-elusive goal. (You had to have read our first volume to understand). I fleetingly thought I would write about that. As it stands, I am sitting on the last night before the deadline, writing about yet another unwelcomed intruder in my body, lupus being the first.

On the day after Christmas 2017, I had a medical emergency that required immediate and invasive surgery. I was cut open from my pelvis to my sternum, and a mass was found. Two days later, I learned it was malignant. The tears did not come for me until 15

A History with God

days later, on the day of my PET scan.[1] I walked into the scanning room, and the machine seemed so ominous and cold. It broke me emotionally knowing that the surgery may not have gotten it all, that there may be more cancer. The technicians were very kind; they let me get my full ugly cry out.

Now admittedly, I am a bit of a hypochondriac! My imagination ran wild in that moment of facing the scanning machine. I posit that I am allowed some leeway considering that I have experienced a staph infection which led to 18 operations on my hands and wrists, a cardiac arrest on the operating table which took me completely out for 20 minutes, and four and a half years on dialysis. Now that you have read that, I'm sure you too agree that I've earned the right to have some hypochondriac tendencies!

Well, as I faced the scanning machine, I figured that the reason I had been so forgetful was because the cancer was in my brain, obviously. I figured the reason my joints hurt so badly intermittently was because the cancer was in my bones, obviously. Boy, was I ever glad to learn that I was just becoming an "older" person when the results came back.

The PET scan revealed that there is additional cancer, but it is all localized to one location—neither of which is my brain or my bones, thankfully. As I sit writing, I am halfway through my treatments. I am initially being treated with Rituxan, a drug familiar to most chronic lupus patients. If the Rituxan proves unsuccessful in eradicating the cancer, then I will undergo intensive chemotherapy.

Being a woman of faith, I am trusting God to work yet another healing miracle in my body. I have already experienced the Lord performing so many miraculous things that not even my doctors

---

[1] A PET scan, also called positron emission tomography scan, is described by the National Cancer Institute as a "procedure in which a small amount of radioactive glucose (sugar) is injected into a vein, and a scanner is used to make detailed, computerized pictures of areas inside the body where the glucose is taken up."

Fighting Lupus Battles

could fully explain. I know God never changes, and if He healed me before, He can do it again. I am neither discouraged nor fearful. I have a history with God, and He is my healer still.

Commentary by Dr. Rosalind Ramsey-Goldman
Lupus patients have a slight increased risk of certain cancers, so it is important to not only keep up with regular appointments for lupus care, but also for routine health care including recommended screening for cancer. In this case, a medical problem led to an operation where the cancer was found. So it is also important to seek care for a new or changing complaint.

The Other Side of Fear: Living My Life Despite Lupus

Ashley Chappell-Rice

> "Pregnancy, when lupus is not controlled, can be risky for both mother and baby. In this case, lupus became even more active during pregnancy and could even flare more after the pregnancy is over. In this case, the placenta separated from the womb too soon, resulting in blood loss which was life threatening for both mother and child. Unfortunately the baby did not survive, but this mother is strong and has found the will to live, the drive to improve lupus awareness, and the mission to highlight the importance of research because we need better treatments for lupus."
>
> —Dr. Rosalind Ramsey-Goldman in
> *Fighting Lupus Battles: Hope for a Cure*

EVERYTHING WE WANT is on the other side of fear. I remember that during one of my appointments my rheumatologist gave me a look of great concern. She said, "You want to have another baby? Are you afraid after what happened the last time?"

Without thinking, I responded with my heart. "I want a baby more than I am afraid." She nodded with understanding.

You're probably wondering what she meant by the last time. This is what happened the last time. Four months into my last pregnancy, I was diagnosed with lupus and started seeing my rheumatologist. At seven months, I had a placental abruption, which

Fighting Lupus Battles

means the placenta detaches from the uterus prematurely. We lost our son, whom we named Zion, and I almost lost my life.

After that tragedy, my rheumatologist strongly recommended that I wait at least two years before trying to get pregnant again. She wanted to observe my course with lupus before determining if pregnancy would even be an option for me. It was such a big tragedy for us. Everyone was so fearful of what might happen to me. My doctors, my family, and my friends wrote off the idea of my having another baby. Immediately after it happened, I didn't think about having another baby either. So many things changed all at once. At that time, my concern centered on healing from the loss and finding a new normal.

While nothing could ever replace my precious baby Zion, my desire to have another baby began to creep back into my mind. You see, I had only been married one year when all of that happened. We really wanted Zion. Experiencing the tragic loss of him didn't erase the desire to expand our family. At the time, we had one daughter already, and many people told me to just be satisfied with her. I was, but she wanted a sibling, and I wanted more children. To be honest, it weighed heavily on me as a woman to hear that I couldn't have any more children, especially when my body had already lost one. It just seemed like all hope was gone. On one hand, we had to bury our son. On the other hand, we were dealing with burying the possibility of giving birth to more children. For two years I tried to discuss having more children with my doctor, but she was serious. She was against risking my life no matter how persistent I was.

Another doctor read about what I went through the last time and told me I was crazy. But one thing I have learned to ask myself is, *if I live my life in fear, what life would I have?* Yes, lupus is scary. Yes, lupus has caused me pain and loss. Every day with every breath I'm reminded that I am sick. I have lost so much in the past: my home, my car, my

The Other Side of Fear

job, money, my son, and I almost lost my life. But I refuse to let fear stand in my way.

One day at my appointment, I was talking with a physician who was doing a post-doctoral fellowship at my rheumatologist's practice. Before leaving to meet with my rheumatologist, he asked if there was anything else that I wanted to discuss. Jokingly, I said, "Well, I want to get pregnant." He was new to me and didn't really know the history of my asking my rheumatologist about getting pregnant. I didn't want him to really go back and tell her what I said. I was sure she was tired of hearing me ask about having a baby. They came back in the room together. She sat down, looked at me, and said, "So you really want to have another baby." You see, she is a doctor who really listens to her patients. I believe she saw my sadness and desire to have another baby. I believe she understood my position. What good would I be "lupus healthy" if I was sad on the inside? To my surprise, she finally said, "OK."

I couldn't believe it. From that point, she and many other doctors reviewed all my risks. My obstetrics and gynecology (OB/GYN) doctors who specialized in pregnancy and childbirth even arranged an appointment where they only talked about all the scary things that could happen. Immediately, my husband and I tried to get pregnant. But nothing in life is that easy, especially when you have lupus. A month later, I found out I had a lung disease and would have to start seeing a pulmonologist. During my first appointment with the pulmonologist, I told her I was trying to get pregnant. She told me she wanted me to wait three years. She also wanted to increase my prednisone from the five mg that I was taking to forty mg. I cried on the spot. It felt like I took one step forward only to take ten steps back. Through tears I told her I couldn't wait. She listened and agreed. You see, wanting to get pregnant was not just about what could happen once I was pregnant, it also made my medical treatment very limited as far as the medications I could take. That made my doctors' job even harder than it already was.

As months turned into years, I was putting off medication and treatments that I couldn't have due to my wanting to get pregnant. Here I was waiting to get pregnant only to find now I was struggling with infertility. Every month when my period came, I became sad because I felt like a failure. Some months my period was late. I would get excited, only to be let down when it showed up. I saw doctors who specialize in fertility, and they were not able to determine why I wasn't getting pregnant. I was even considering getting fertility treatment. The fertility specialists requested written approval from my rheumatologist, which I figured might be a problem. It had been almost three years since my rheumatologist said I could get pregnant. With that length of time, the recent diagnosis of lung disease, and hospitalizations, I wasn't certain if she would still agree.

In the meantime, I decided to try other methods. I arranged acupuncture appointments, I began to eat healthier, and I established a strenuous workout schedule. My first acupuncture visit was definitely mind-opening. After two sessions, my period was late. I didn't even get excited because that had happened many times before, and I had ended up being disappointed. I figured I had become irregular and wasn't tracking it right. Just to be sure I wasn't pregnant, I decided to take a pregnancy test. I didn't want to work out too hard if I was pregnant. I was so sure I was going to be disappointed. I felt that I was being irrational just spending the money on the test. But it's always when you least expect something that it happens. Finally, after so many times of getting negatives and things being taken away from me due to lupus, the pregnancy test was positive. I was pregnant; I was so happy.

Immediately, I followed up with my doctors and the high-risk pregnancy team. As time progressed during my pregnancy, I began to get nervous. I started having flashbacks of what hap-

The Other Side of Fear

pened the last time and felt anxious at times. But a part of me felt brave. Brave for doing what most people wouldn't. I felt brave for not letting my past or lupus stop me.

Most of my pregnancy was normal. I saw my OB/GYN doctors often and continued to follow up with my lupus and lung doctors. I found out I was having a girl, and from what we could tell, she was healthy. I was secure in the idea that I would have a cesarean surgery, also known as C-section, to deliver her. I thought it would be safest. I thought it was my only option. During my last delivery, I had an emergency C-section. I was cut vertically on the outer layers of my abdomen. Around five or six months into my pregnancy, my doctors found out that despite my vertical scar on my abdomen, my uterus was actually cut horizontally, making it possible for me to have a VBAC (vaginal birth after cesarean). Having the opportunity to choose between C-section and vaginal delivery made me more nervous. What if I chose the wrong thing and something happened? Both options had risks.

I was also pressuring my doctors to schedule an early delivery. I believed that an early delivery would help to prevent what happened the last time. I was sure things would go better with an early delivery. But the high-risk team refused and said that as long as everything was going fine, they couldn't schedule an early delivery.

Another concern was getting to the hospital in time. You see, I live an hour away from my hospital, so I had concerns about not getting there in time. The last time, I delivered at a local hospital, and things didn't end up well. I didn't want that to happen again. So a month and a half before my due date, I stayed downtown, closer to my hospital. About a week into my stay, I woke up one morning to find my water had broken. I couldn't believe it. Just like I wanted, she was coming exactly one month early and without them having to induce me. Upon arrival at the hospital, I was all set to go for my C-section when the doctor came in and reminded me that during one of my visits, I expressed some feelings about the delivery. In that visit, I was asked if I would have a C-section or vaginal delivery. I responded that if I went into natural labor like my water breaking, I would just have her naturally. If not, I would get a C-section.

Let me tell you, my own words came back to bite me in the butt. I really didn't want to do a vaginal delivery. I didn't believe I could push with the breathing problems I have due to lupus. I was actually surprised that they thought I could do it. I was afraid of my C-section scar opening up. More importantly, I was afraid that my baby could die during the labor process. Even though the doctors told me recovery from surgery would be harder on my body due to lupus, I was more concerned about the baby. I was scared to make the wrong decision.

The doctors spent a great deal of time reassuring me that the baby would be fine. They explained that trying a vaginal delivery was actually better for her because it would help squeeze fluid from her lungs. It would make it easier for her to breathe.

I realized I didn't come all this way to be scared. Plus, they offered me a turkey sandwich, and I was hungry. If I had the C-section, I would have to wait to eat. I took the sandwich. I was having my baby vaginally.

I was given an epidural, and it really helped with the pain and actually allowed me to breathe a lot easier than I had expected. The nurse and staff were amazing. I felt so powerful, brave, and strong when it came time to push her out. Finally, my body was doing something right. In that moment, the doctors and I were surprised that I didn't have any pain. The doctor kept saying, "Take your time if you need it." I think I surprised her. I pushed my baby out with five pushes. I was so proud of my body and myself. For once it felt like my mind and body were on the same page for something. The best thing was hearing my baby's strong cry. They put her in my arms. She was here. I gave birth to a healthy baby girl.

The Other Side of Fear

I look back over the years I spent waiting for her. I see all the things that could have stopped me—the tears, the fears, and the doubts. I realize that having my baby girl is the definition of living your life despite lupus. This is what it means to learn to live with lupus. It's realizing that your life isn't filled with the word "no" all the time. You don't have to stop wanting to live. You can have a regular life; you just may have to go about it a different way. It may be harder. You may have to wait, but you will get there. Just be brave enough to live. That's why we are called lupus warriors.

Commentary by Dr. Rosalind Ramsey-Goldman

Since lupus affects primarily young women, questions related to pregnancy are important topics to discuss with your doctor. The questions may include: Can I become pregnant? What will happen to my baby if I have lupus? What will happen to me if I become pregnant? Can I take medication when pregnant, and which ones are safe for the baby? Working with a team of specialists to control lupus for the mother gives the best chance for a good outcome for mother and baby.

Fortunate and Grateful
Tari Ambler

In the first book, Fighting Lupus Battles: Hope for a Cure, *the title of Tari's story is "Armed with Hope and Knowledge". She wrote, "I decided, with God's help, I was going to manage this illness and do what I could to live normally. I knew I would have to keep a positive attitude if I was going to be successful." I salute Tari for continuing to have a positive attitude, a necessary weapon in our lupus battles.*

I HAVE BEEN FORTUNATE to be doing very well physically, and I am thankful that my lupus is still in remission. I have enjoyed being an active volunteer at my church and in the community. Facilitating a lupus support group from 2002 through 2017 has also been a joy. I'm extremely grateful to God that I feel well and have the energy to enjoy life and to help others. I've always tried to have hope, even when my journey was difficult. Now I am experiencing good health, and I pray God will continue to bless me with good health in the years to come.

Commentary by Dr. Rosalind Ramsey-Goldman
Being involved in support groups is one way to help others while helping yourself too.

Just Like That: Another Chance at Life

Ivy M. Douglas

On July 5, 2016, I received a phone call from my doctor stating that my kidney function had dropped to fifteen percent. She told me I had to make a decision as soon as possible—dialysis or kidney transplant. Of course, I didn't want to do either, but I had no other choice. My kidney function was decreasing daily.

I had an opportunity to visit a dialysis center. I sat there looking at the patients and seeing the horrible side effects of dialysis. Many of the patients were depressed and complained about joint and muscle stiffness. Some were even throwing up. I couldn't believe how something that's supposed to help could bring so much harm to you. After leaving there, all I could do was cry and pray. I just couldn't see myself going through that. I didn't want to ever experience dialysis.

So, my next choice was to have a kidney transplant. I connected with a hospital and started the transplantation process. I had many blood tests as well as meetings with doctors and social workers. I was introduced to the packet that I needed to share with potential donors. Then I was placed on the kidney transplant registry as a recipient. I sent text messages to friends and family members asking them to be my donors. Ten people responded and went through the process. Many of them were declined due to weight or because their blood type didn't match mine. There was one who was a perfect match—my childhood friend, but she lived in Mississippi. The doctors preferred working with one of my potential donors who lived closer to Chicago.

Fighting Lupus Battles

My hospital had a program where they cross-matched donors with cooperating transplantation centers. So, if one of my donors matched a recipient from a cooperating center, and one of their donors matched me, the two cooperating centers would switch kidneys. Unfortunately, that didn't work for me. So, we were back to my childhood friend. She came to Chicago several times to meet with the social worker and the surgery team. Once she finished the process, our date for the surgery was set for September 2, 2016.

On the big day, we arrived at the hospital early that morning for our prep. She went into surgery first. Her surgery lasted about three hours. Then it was my turn. Boy, was I nervous! This was my first time having major surgery. My surgery lasted longer than expected, but it went well. My doctors explained that my new kidney was functioning at eighty-five percent. My friend was released to go home the next day, but I had to be monitored in the hospital for several days after surgery.

Upon my release from the hospital, I was told to expect a six-week healing process. I was given a list of appointments and a bag of new pills—eight per day, to be exact. I was already taking seven pills a day. So, that meant I'd have to manage fifteen meds daily. One thing they didn't tell me was how much pain I might experience. I took so many pain pills just to rest. I was at the doctor's office every week for the full six-week recovery period for follow-up and blood work. During my recovery, I ended up with a kidney infection that put me in the hospital for a week. While I was in the hospital, I also suffered obstruction in my lungs. So we had another problem that required more testing and a longer hospital stay. I was not a happy camper.

After being released from the hospital, I was back on my healing journey. I continued going to my weekly doctor appointments and having my weekly blood draws. Medication side effects led to the need to make many changes in prescriptions. So, I was still adjusting to my new medications. The pain began to subside, and I was

Just Like That: Another Chance at Life

able to rest a little better. My scar started to show some signs of healing. I was beginning to feel like myself again.

Then it was time for one of my three biopsies. My six-month biopsy entailed doctors taking three snips from my kidney. It was an in-and-out procedure, unlike pre-transplantation biopsies when I had to stay in the hospital for days. It took a couple of days for the pain to go away. While recovering from my biopsy, I developed a high fever (103.1 degrees). I let it linger for days before going to the hospital. The doctors ran test after test trying to find out what was going on. After two days of testing, the doctors realized I had internal bleeding. They explained to me that my artery had been clipped. When I asked how that happened, of course they were hesitant to tell me. Finally, they broke down and said it happened during the biopsy. So, I had been bleeding internally for two weeks. If I had waited any longer I would have died. I had to have an emergency procedure to have a stent placed in my artery to stop the bleeding. After surgery, I had to have a blood transfusion to replace all the blood I had lost. I was very hesitant about doing the blood transfusion because I had never had that procedure done before, but I knew I needed it.

Almost seven months into my recovery journey, doctors informed me that my kidney function had decreased to fifty percent due to damage it had sustained over the past couple months, and it was all out of my control. I was not happy about that news at all, especially since I knew that people weren't just handing out kidneys. I went through an emotional journey. I had so many mixed feelings after all I had been through. I wanted to find a lawyer and sue the hospital and the doctor. I tried, but I wasn't successful. Many of the lawyers told me that the malpractice laws had changed; the battle wasn't worth the fight.

Just when I thought I was in the clear, doctors called to tell me I had a virus called CMV. According to the Centers for Disease Control and Prevention, CMV or cytomegalovirus is a common virus that infects people of all ages, but it can cause serious health problems for people with weakened immune systems. When I asked where the CMV came from, they informed me that it came with the kidney. I asked why I wasn't informed about this prior to my transplant. My doctor said that he weighed the risk factors. He determined that having the transplant was most important, and CMV could be treated.

Even though I didn't want to take any more pills, I started the treatment right away. While going through the treatment, I developed a low white blood cell count, and my immune system was compromised. As a result, I had to have weekly neutropenia shots to build up my cell count. With all that going on, I felt I was almost forced to live in a bubble. The possibility of picking up germs caused the need for me to be extremely cautious as I went places and met with people. So, my social life decreased, and I didn't get out much with friends or family. Wearing a mask was embarrassing for me. People tended to stare and give all kinds of looks. I hated that, but I knew it was all for my benefit.

After all of that, I went back to my regular routine of traveling, working, and enjoying life as I knew it before transplantation. Then I received another phone call from my doctor. He informed me that my kidney function had dropped to 23 percent, showing signs of rejection. Another biopsy needed to be done immediately. I was very nervous, especially after what happened during the last biopsy. The biopsy confirmed signs of rejection. Trying to save my kidney, we started an aggressive treatment—three weeks of steroids, delivered intravenously.

The steroid dosage started at 160mg and decreased weekly by 20mg. With doses that high, I started experiencing side effects right away. The side effects included a balloon face, weight loss, acne, swelling in my feet and ankles, and many others. Once I was finished with the IV treatment, I started taking steroids in pill form. I started at 100mg and reduced it by 20mg daily until I was down to 10mg. My kidney reacted to the treatment as expected. My kidney function increased to 48 percent, more than double what it had

Just Like That: Another Chance at Life

been. My kidney was finally stable, and the doctors decreased the steroids down to 5mg. With that change, my kidney function started to decrease again. My immune system became more compromised, and I ended up back in the hospital. That time it was for the flu and pneumonia. Being back in the hospital was not what I was looking for. I spent several days there, having to endure one test after another as doctors tried to develop a treatment plan.

It's been a rocky road. I endured the biopsies, the transplant surgery, changes in the medications and the side effects, the many hospitalizations, and the constant blood draws (sticks). Then there were the doctor's mistakes that almost cost me my kidney. If I had known I would have to go through so much with my decision to have the transplant, I probably would have gone a different route.

Currently, I am still fighting to save my kidney. It is functioning at 23 percent again. I am still going for my weekly blood draws. Doctors began talking about repeating the transplantation process. They explained to me that this happens with a lot of patients; many of them must have more than one transplant. But repeating transplantation is not something I want to do.

I need this kidney to function for me over the next 51 years because I am looking to live until I am ninety. To help my kidney fight, I have made changes in many areas of my life, especially with eating habits. I have also started talking to my body and my kidney daily, using declarations regarding healing. I am praying and believing that God will turn my kidney function around. I was BLESSED to get this gift of another chance at life, so I am going to do my best to keep it.

Fighting Lupus Battles

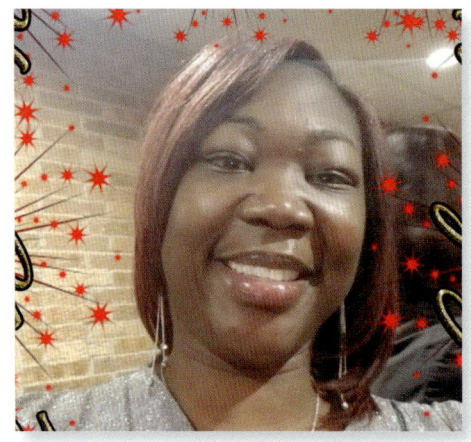

Ivy Douglas

Commentary by Dr. Rosalind Ramsey-Goldman

Kidney problems are the most common serious problem for lupus patients. When the kidneys do not work properly, challenging decisions need to be made regarding what to do for renal replacement—dialysis or transplant. Sometimes even in the best of circumstances, things do not always go smoothly. Lupus patients are fighters dealing with adversity every day.

Fighting and Hoping for the Best

Helena Fields

This year marks my 25th anniversary. No, I am not married, although I imagine having lupus is similar to having a nagging husband. Just like a marriage, having lupus consists of ups and downs. In the past, I focused on the downs; however, this is the year I am determined to have more of a positive outlook. I figured that if I made it this far I could keep going and try harder to make the journey easier. There was a time when I did not believe I would survive five years, but here I am. I have learned a lot about myself over the years as it pertains to my health. However, it wasn't until last year that I realized I needed to fully accept that I have lupus and that it isn't going away.

Last year, I decided it was time for a new rheumatologist. There wasn't anything wrong with my old one, except the fact that she was connected to a teaching hospital. She wasn't the issue, but her residents were. At each visit, there would be a new resident, and I'd have to tell my story over again. I always felt like I was under a microscope. I am such an interesting case for them because my labs show that I'm near death, but I appear fine. I also have to mention that in addition to seeing a rheumatologist, I also see an internist, nephrologist, hematologist, gynecologist, and psychologist pretty often. My patience for doctors' visits is thin, so I really didn't want to be bothered with new residents each time.

I searched online for a new rheumatologist. I came across a doctor who had given some educational seminars to help people cope with their diagnosis, and I made an appointment to see her. Upon

Fighting Lupus Battles

the first visit, she had already reviewed my lab work that I had sent to her from the previous doctor. She told me she wasn't pleased with my condition. I told her I wasn't pleased either. I only had a period of remission once since I was diagnosed, and that took place 13 years ago! The only time when I exhibited no signs or symptoms of having lupus was while I was pregnant. Other than that, there has always been something wrong. There was always some pain or symptom that reminded me lupus was there.

When I met the new rheumatologist last year, she asked me a question that no other doctor ever asked me before. She asked, "Have you fully accepted that you have lupus?" At that point, I couldn't stop the tears from flowing. It had been 24 years since the diagnosis, and the truth is I hadn't really accepted it. I viewed myself as having some limitations, but I would either try to ignore lupus or fix it. I couldn't accept that I had to learn to live with it. I had spent so much of my life in doctors' offices and hospital beds. I hated taking medications. I just wanted to be cured. I wanted to feel normal. I didn't want to be restricted from doing the things I love. I wanted to play in the sun. I didn't want to feel different.

I know there is no magic potion that will cure me, but there are some things that will assist me in living my best life. The most important things I found are self-care, lots of rest, and a healthy diet. It seems like a simple solution, but it is often difficult to maintain. Self-care includes many things. In particular, it involves living a life with as little stress as possible and taking care of yourself. A regular day for a healthy person is filled with stressors such as work, family, financial concerns, etc. Now add in some health issues like chronic pain and unexplained illnesses. I am a special education teacher and a doctoral student, but foremost I am a single parent to a teen. Therefore, stress is a part of my daily life. I try my best to balance it, but it is not an easy task.

Considering all that I have on my plate, you can pretty much figure out that I do not get much sleep. Even when I do fall asleep, I wake up at least twice each night to use the bathroom. There are times

Fighting and Hoping for the Best

when my body decides it's going to rest regardless of whether I want it to or not. There have been days when I couldn't get out of the bed because my legs and arms were stiff and sore. It is on those days I struggle physically and mentally. I don't like to appear weak. People, even those closest to me, think I'm being lazy or just avoiding work. The reality is I have neglected getting the required rest for so long that I just can't keep going. I had to learn not to care what others thought. I have to pay attention to what my body needs. So if it needs rest then I rest.

The other thing I have noticed that helps is when I eat healthier. This seems like a no-brainer, but I am an emotional eater. Nothing makes me feel better on a stressful day than a piece of cake and some cheese fries. I am a foodie. I like trying new restaurants and recipes. My time is limited, so I have eaten a lot of dinners in my car straight out of the drive-thru. I know these are bad habits, and I am trying to change. I had a rude awakening the last time I was in the hospital in August 2016. I have stage 4 kidney disease, and I am a few steps away from dialysis. While in the hospital, I was on a renal diet. There were so many food items that I couldn't have due to my disease. I realized how poor my diet was and how I was possibly making myself sicker due to my horrible choices. I vowed to make a change. My diet has improved, but there is still much more work to do.

I wanted this year to be special. I was finally ready to make positive changes in order to live my best life. My intentions are good, but each time I take three steps forward only to get knocked twenty steps back. I started counting calories using My Fitness Pal. I just needed something to hold me accountable for what I was eating. I had been sticking to eating between the hours of 10 a.m. and 6 p.m., and I was also going to bed earlier. The later I'm awake, the more likely I'll want a snack. I was getting ready to start working out three times a week when I noticed that I was dizzy and light-headed. It was a familiar issue; my blood count was too low. I had an appointment with the nephrologist coming up in January 2017,

Fighting Lupus Battles

so I waited until the appointment for him to confirm what I already knew. However, this time it was lower than it had been in years. My hemoglobin was 6.1 g/dL, which is about half of what it should be.

I had to get a blood transfusion immediately. I was also told to limit my activity. I needed Procrit injections. However, my insurance has been reluctant to cover them. The Procrit injections are expensive, and the doctors want to try cheaper alternatives such as iron. The problem is that I do not have an iron deficiency; my kidney just doesn't produce red blood cells. I'm fatigued and weak all the time. I've started to develop worse headaches. I try not to complain about my symptoms because I don't want to have to go to the hospital. I just want to get better.

This has been my life with lupus. It's been a constant battle, filled with highs and lows. I'm at a low point, but I am striving to go higher. I have to believe that things will get better. It is difficult at times to be optimistic, but what is the alternative? I'd rather hope for better days than to wallow in sadness, so I'll keep fighting and hoping for the best.

Commentary by Dr. Rosalind Ramsey-Goldman

Learning to live with and accept that you have a chronic illness is one of the many hardships confronting people with lupus. Having kidney disease is one of the most serious problems with lupus. Taking control of the parts of your life that you can impact, such as being more physically active, are actions you can take to feel better. Get advice from your healthcare providers on how to live better with lupus.

Lupus Lessons

Patricia L. Sanders

Patricia is my niece who was diagnosed with lupus a few years ago. Pat wrote in my first book, "Though my sister fought like a champion, she lost her battle with lupus in 1997 at the age of thirty-two". This is what Pat wants to share about her life since the 2015 publication of Fighting Lupus Battles: Hope for a Cure.

MY LIFE SINCE 2015 has been up and down. There have been good days and bad ones, especially with sinus problems. When I was diagnosed in 2011, I was advised to meet with my rheumatologist four times a year and to take two pills (Plaquenil) every day. Now I only have to see my doctor twice a year for lupus. The medication schedule is to take two pills one day and one pill the next day. I'm looking forward to the time when I will have to see my doctor only once a year and my medication is cut to one pill per day, or ideally none at all.

I have learned so much since I was diagnosed. I learned that educating myself about lupus is very important. Through education, I gained a better understanding of the disease, its potential impact on my life, and ways to take care of myself. I have learned that scheduling and keeping visits with my doctor, learning as much as I can about my disease, exercising, maintaining a proper diet, and taking my medication as prescribed all work together to help keep my lupus in check. I have a name for my medication—the aspirin of lupus. I see it as a barrier to keep anything in my blood from causing more damage than what is there. It helps in allowing

Fighting Lupus Battles

the positive to move within my body, especially into the lupus-infested joints.

My prayer is that one day, lupus will no longer be the headache of my life. It causes so many families to want to give up because of the pain, the medication, and knowing that you have done all you can. Not learning the facts about lupus can make one feel helpless. One fact that my doctor shared with me is that since I was diagnosed, lupus research has made much progress, especially within the past few years. I am glad to hear and see that the world is paying more attention to lupus and is starting to understand that this chronic disease has no boundaries. My advice is to pay attention to your body. If you are having any lupus-like symptoms, take the time to see a doctor and ask to be evaluated for lupus.

My most important lesson was to keep a close relationship with God through prayer, faith, love, and belief. I feel I must remember that God's Word is a lamp unto my feet. That Word/lamp directs my path and orders my steps. I see lupus as an evil weapon and believe that it shall not prosper against me. I've learned to be cool, as the kids say, and to take one day at a time. My faith is strong, and I believe that if we keep searching for a cure, it will happen.

Commentary by Dr. Rosalind Ramsey-Goldman
Learning as much as you can about lupus and your medications is one way to cope with a chronic illness such as lupus. Understanding why it is important to keep up with the doctor's visits and taking the medication will increase the chances of you getting better. Over time, if all goes well, you will need to see the doctor less often and might be able to take less medication, while being able to lead a fulfilling life.

Vision–Living a Life Without Lupus

Sarah Spadoni, CVT

IT'S A GLOOMY day in April of 2017 when I walk into the outpatient center at the hospital, with my boyfriend and my mother by my side. So many worries are going through my mind, and the only thing that makes me feel somewhat calm is knowing that I have the best support around.

Today I am having a new procedure done. The attendant takes me up to my room and gives me a gown for me to change into. I have a little time alone to breathe and take in what is about to happen. My stomach is in knots. I have to keep telling myself, *No matter what happens, I will get through it.*

The nurse comes back in and asks me many questions about all my medical conditions, medications, and allergies. She then places an IV (a needle or tube inserted into a vein) and starts me on fluids to rehydrate me since I fasted all night. We sit there in a weird silence. No one wants to talk about what is about to happen. I focus in on the television and the small talk between my boyfriend and mother, who are meeting for the first time. A couple hours later, it's time. A volunteer comes in with a wheelchair to take me down for the procedure. I am on the verge of a panic attack. I have to keep reminding myself, *It isn't going to hurt that bad, and no matter what happens I'm going to be OK*. We enter a very small room that has a bed that is half the size of the room, a counter with a sink, cabinets, a rather large ultrasound machine, monitoring equipment, and three other people beside myself. They take my vitals and explain the procedure. They say I should only feel a little pressure so I don't need anesthesia. I'm worried that I won't be under for this, but they try to reassure me by telling me that I won't feel anything. As I lie on my stomach in this tiny and cramped room, they start giving me some medication through my IV. I start to relax, and all my worries start to fade away. It is actually comforting, being able to talk during the procedure. They talk me through everything and are actually done within a few minutes. They check the incision to make sure I don't have any extra bleeding. They advise me to rest for the next few hours without moving around and to spend the rest of the day relaxing. I'm done with my kidney biopsy.

I can't help but check MyChart, an online system I use to communicate with my doctors, every day for the results of the biopsy. Finally, the results post on MyChart. Immediately, the tears start to flow as I focus on the words *"consistent with lupus nephritis."* Of course, I have no clue what this means. I read the pathology report over and over again and start searching Google. Getting information from Google and talking with the doctor allow me to gather that, yes I do have lupus nephritis—classes III and V. Basically that means that lupus is attacking my kidneys to the point where they aren't functioning properly. I always had a feeling a day like this would come.

My lupus journey started around 2007. It took me three different doctors and three years to get an accurate diagnosis. I started off with fatigue and saw myself as having a mild case of lupus. I should not have looked at any disease like that, especially lupus. It made it seem like it was not serious and sometimes made me overlook some of my symptoms. Unfortunately, I got to a point in my fight with lupus that I gave up really fighting for myself. I should have pushed the doctors years ago to look further into the elevation of protein in my urine. I should have fought for myself more.

After I was diagnosed with lupus nephritis, my doctors developed a treatment plan to help prevent more damage to my kidneys.

Vision–Living a Life Without Lupus

They prescribed a stronger immunosuppressant, vitamin D, medications for blood pressure, prednisone, and a handful of other medications and supplements. I couldn't have alcohol or NSAIDs (nonsteroidal anti-inflammatory drugs) and had to be careful with other over-the-counter medications. I started seeing the nephrologist and rheumatologist every six to twelve weeks for rechecks. My kidneys have been improving slowly. I do, however, think I will always have some scar tissue on my kidneys.

Now I have so many different symptoms and related disease processes. My symptoms include fatigue, joint and muscle pain, joint swelling, connective tissue inflammation (tendinitis and bursitis), urinary tract issues, stomach pain, headaches, nose and mouth sores, vision problems, bruising, low platelets, fainting, dizziness, abnormal autoimmune blood panels, and I'm sure so much more. I have been diagnosed with diseases like Raynaud's disease,[1] Sjogren's syndrome,[2] allergies, and lupus nephritis (inflammation of the kidney).

I've been hospitalized for fainting and having chest pain. We still haven't discovered the reasons I have these issues. I end up just chalking everything up to lupus.

My job as a veterinary technician is very strenuous and exhausting, not only physically but also emotionally. I fight to push myself through the exhaustion, pain, and headaches that I have daily. Every morning is a struggle to get out of bed. All I want to do is stay in bed and sleep, so I press the snooze button multiple times. After about twenty minutes, I force myself out of bed at the last

---

[1] MedlinePlus defines Raynaud's disease as "a rare disorder of the blood vessels, usually in the fingers and toes. It causes the blood vessels to narrow when you are cold or feeling stressed. When this happens, blood can't get to the surface of the skin and the affected areas turn white and blue."

[2] MedlinePlus describes Sjögren's syndrome as "a disease that affects the glands that make moisture. It most often causes dryness in the mouth and eyes. It can also lead to dryness in other places that need moisture, such as the nose, throat, and skin."

Fighting Lupus Battles

second and stumble to the bathroom. I get ready as quickly as I can because I'm always running late. No matter how much sleep I get, I NEVER feel rested. I'm constantly yawning throughout the day.

After work, I am drained and often have to take a nap. On days when I nap, I have to set an alarm; otherwise, I might nap for four hours. If I'm not napping, I am resting on the couch. Thinking about how much time I spend relaxing or sleeping is actually depressing. I try never to let it overcome me, but there are times where I need to break down and cry.

Lupus has made me not care too much about how I look. I barely wear any make up and almost never do my hair. Showering is even more exhausting, and I always save that for at night. I even put it off when I can. It takes a lot of effort to wash everything. All I want to do is sit down and let the water pour down on me and not move.

When I do too much or have overwhelming stress, my body screams at me. When this happens I start to flare up a little. The exhaustion gets worse, and my body starts to feel like it's on fire. I have such random symptoms when this occurs. Most of the time my joints become painful and swollen. My muscles ache and burn. My headache gets worse, and I start to become nauseated. I get sores that spread over a large area inside and outside of my nose. They are bright red and sometimes ooze and bleed. They are itchy and very painful at times and can last for weeks.

The times when I am in a big lupus flare are the worst, and I can't do anything. My body screams ten times more than before, and the pain seems like it is never going to end. It feels like every inch of me is on fire or broken. Every touch and movement hurts. The pain is so unbearable and constant during this time; no matter what I do, it never lets up. I try to get as much rest as possible, but that's so hard to do because of the constant and excruciating pain I'm in all over my body. During these times with the constant throbbing pain, I just break down and cry.

Vision–Living a Life Without Lupus

These are the times when I feel like lupus has won and taken over my body. Being tough is the only option I have though. No one ever said this would be easy, but no one ever told me it would be this hard either. It is so hard to describe the different types of pain I feel daily. I wish I could explain it so people could understand what I'm going through and would cut me some slack if I'm not myself.

Lupus is definitely a rollercoaster ride; you never know minute to minute how you may feel. Lupus patients need to know their lab results and discover what's not normal for them. Frequent blood and urine tests are so important in lupus patients. The results could give clues as to what is going on in your body and help expose some of the damage lupus is causing. Lupus patients need to be their own advocates and fight for what they need and want.

I wouldn't be able to get through these times if it wasn't for my family and closest friends. They are the ones who constantly push me, joke around, and always tell me they wish they could take away my pain. They support me loud and proud at every Lupus Walk. Also during Lupus Awareness Month in May, they annoy all their friends with information about lupus. I don't know what I would do if I didn't have them as my support team; they mean the world to me. Therefore, I can't give up.

My family and closest friends push me and make me realize there are so many things that I want to do. I want to spread awareness of this nasty disease. I want to figure out a way to go into remission. I want to travel. I want to get married and maybe start a family. I try so hard to not let lupus consume my life. One of these days I will LIVE A LIFE WITHOUT LUPUS.

Fighting Lupus Battles

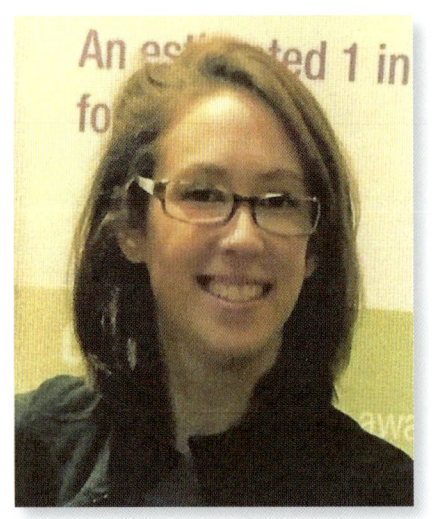

Sarah Spadoni

Commentary by Dr. Rosalind Ramsey-Goldman

Unfortunately, the long journey to getting a diagnosis is not an unusual experience for many patients with lupus. Fatigue is the most common complaint among all lupus patients, and this symptom can be present even if the healthcare provider says all the numbers look good. Treat-to-target is an evolving strategy borrowed from the rheumatologists caring for patients with a related autoimmune condition called rheumatoid arthritis. If you treat early, the target is control of the disease because the goal is to minimize or prevent organ damage. Both patients and doctors need to work together to identify lupus problems early so we can treat sooner and meet our target of no damage as we work towards a cure and a life without lupus.

In Remission: My Life with Lupus, Part II

Kanefus R. Walker

I WROTE THE FIRST part of my lupus story more than two years ago for the 2015 publication of Fighting Lupus Battles: Hope for a Cure. Since then, I have been experiencing some of the busiest times of my life. I have had a full plate. What was I thinking? Was I taking on too much—working on another college degree, joining a sorority, serving in my church, volunteering as leader of my lupus support group, developing plans for opening my own event planning business, and working full-time? Lupus has been pretty stable for me, and I don't want to wake it up.

After thirteen years of being out of school, I chose to pursue a higher college degree. As 2017 came to a close, I was awarded a master's degree in Hospitality and Tourism Management from Roosevelt University in Chicago. That was a huge accomplishment for me. With that done, I began working diligently to open my wedding and event planning business before the end of 2018.

Another huge accomplishment was becoming a part of a sorority, for which I am grateful. After twenty years of waiting for the opportunity, I was initiated into the sorority of my choice. Caring for my community, one of the sorority's core values, is among the top items on my list of priorities. After all, taking care of each other is what God put us here to do.

In addition to earning another college degree and fulfilling my duties in the sorority, I remained active in my church and continued as leader of my support group, The Lupus Connection. Yes, I still led the group, even while pursuing my master's degree. I considered

Fighting Lupus Battles

stepping down from leading the group, but I figured that wouldn't go over too well. Plus we have plenty of work to do with getting the word out about lupus. I still served on the local Lupus Walk committee and was even chosen as the walk's ambassador for two years in a row. That honor allowed me to share my story with more people in the lupus community. The Lupus Connection continues to welcome new faces. When they join the group, some are newly diagnosed; some have been diagnosed for a while. We are still growing. We all need to interact with others who understand the challenges that can come with lupus. I have a great group of people who really come to be supportive of each other.

Even with my busy life, I am still able to manage the lupus. I have had two great doctors throughout my lupus journey. I knew I had help on my side, and that made my lupus battle a bit easier to fight. I lost my first great doctor when she had to relocate due to personal obligations. My second favorite rheumatologist decided to work for another hospital. There I was yet again, feeling vulnerable and afraid the next doctor would not meet my standards. After two years, I am still on the fence about this not-so-new-anymore doctor who is in charge of monitoring my lupus. During each visit, I think more and more about switching hospitals so that I can get my old doctor back. The jury is still out on that decision.

As busy as I have been, the one thing that made the load a bit lighter was that I remained in remission. My current doctor says it's almost like I don't have lupus. My numbers are good, and she has even lowered the dosage on one of my medications. While it makes me happy, I still think about my fellow sisters and brothers who are in the struggle of their lives. For them, I continue to fight. I think about one of my best friends, one of my cousins, one of my former co-workers, and a few of my support group members who lost their battle. It is because of them that I fight. I think about those who are suffering and not accurately diagnosed yet. It is for them that I remain in the trenches and fight.

In Remission: My Life with Lupus, Part II

I am still working full-time. There are even some relocation thoughts swarming around in my head. Maybe I'll get to share that part one day.

I've been overweight most of my life, and it has caused me to not feel very good about myself, to have a low self-esteem about my outward appearance. When I decided to get healthier by exercising and eating better, I began to lose weight, and I started liking what I saw in the mirror for a change. However, losing the weight awakened the lupus, and my initial flare began. I was put on prednisone which brought the weight back on. While I wanted to get back to that girl that I saw in the mirror, the one that I liked, I didn't know if I wanted what came with that. I didn't want to risk bringing on another flare and going through the emotional roller coaster of my weight fluctuating because of the medicines I needed to control the flare.

I haven't gotten the weight thing together yet. After the first flare due to weight loss, it has been a struggle. Part of it has been mental because I don't want to bring on another flare if I should lose too much weight. I don't want the low self-esteem to raise its ugly head now that it is dormant. I have begun to appreciate and in some instances even love myself and what I see in the mirror. I like the new me!

The journey continues, and there is much more work to do. I am blessed for such an assignment God chose to entrust me with. I will keep spreading the word about this disease until I close my eyes into eternity. Sure, it can be frustrating because lupus doesn't get as much notoriety and awareness as other challenging diseases. So we have to keep fighting. I must be encouraged, remain humble, keep a positive attitude, and stay busy fighting. My life with lupus depends on it. My life's story continues and is still being written one flare-free day at a time. Hopefully, one day we can win with a cure.

Fighting Lupus Battles

Commentary by Dr. Rosalind Ramsey-Goldman
Remission is possible, and continuing with meaningful work is doable if you have lupus. This is a message of hope and working towards common goals of living better with lupus and working towards a cure.

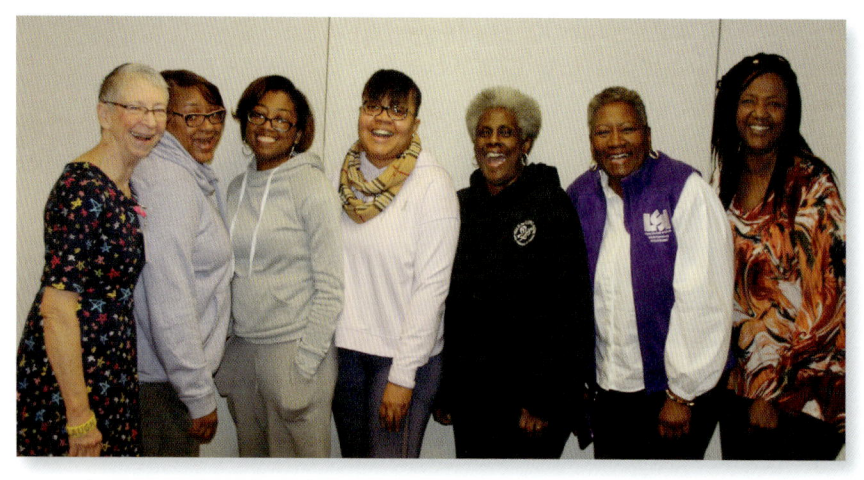

As group leader of The Lupus Connection, Kanefus plans various activities for our support group. On the following page are pictures that were taken at one meeting where Laughologist Kathy O'Brien demonstrated activities that make people laugh.

45

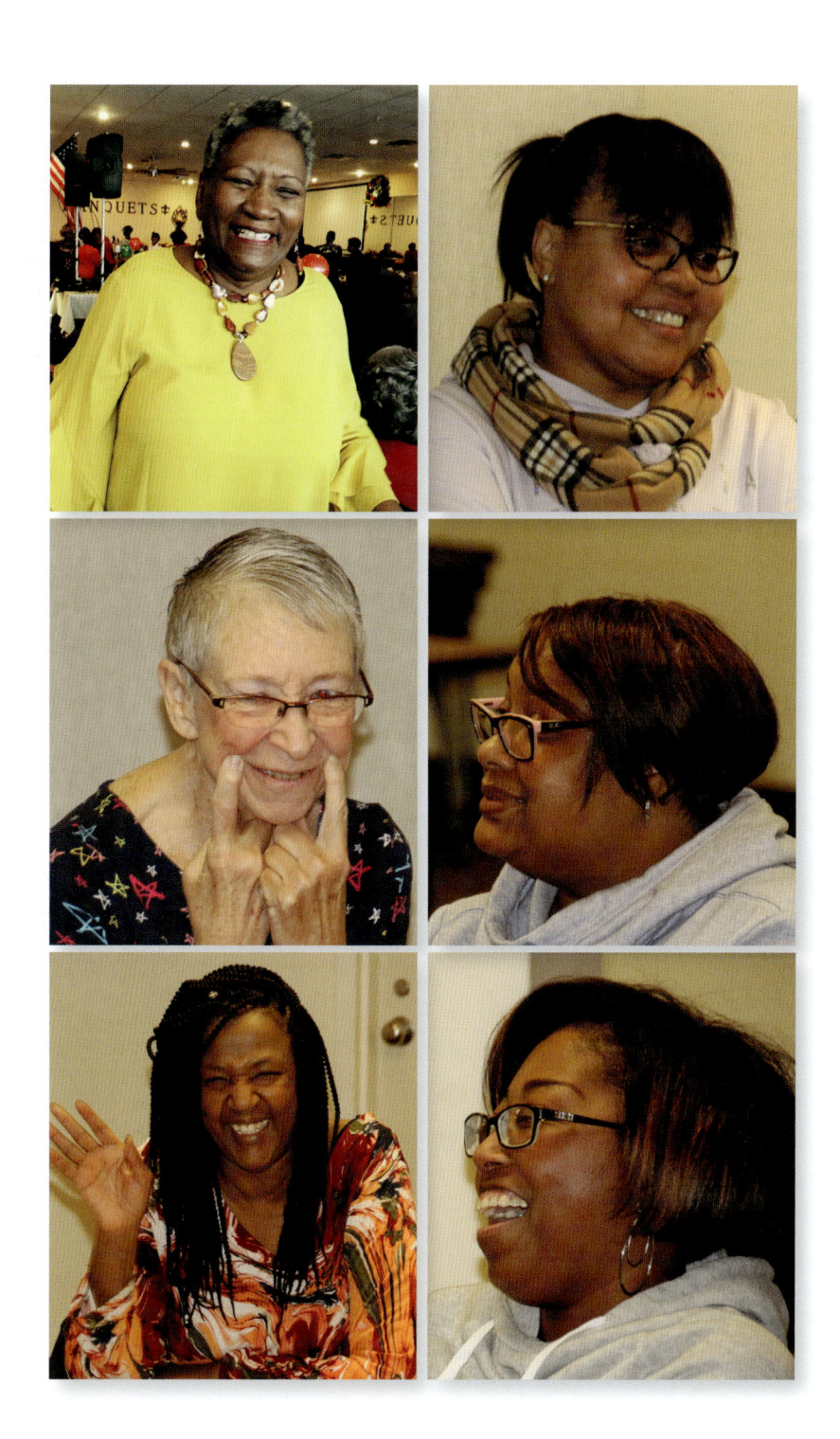

Section II

Journeys of More Lupus Warriors

"**M**OST PEOPLE WITH lupus can live normal lives. Treatment of lupus has improved, and people with the disease are living longer" (ACR—rheumatology.org).

These are tips suggested by the American College of Rheumatology and the National Institutes of Health that may help when living with lupus:

- First, get involved in your care. Learn as much as you can about lupus.

- Form a good relationship with your healthcare team. Work with your doctor to determine a treatment plan. Learn about your medications and what kind of progress to expect.

- Follow your treatment plan religiously by taking all your medications as your doctor prescribes.

- Visit your rheumatologist often to monitor lupus status.

- Pay attention to your body. Learn to recognize the warning signs of having a flare so that you and your doctor might reduce or prevent them.

- Exercise, eat a proper diet, and learn relaxation techniques to help cope with stress. Discuss these with your doctor BEFORE making any changes.

- Develop and maintain a good support system of family, friends, medical professionals, community organizations, faith-based groups, and support groups.
- Avoid excess sun exposure. Sunlight can cause a lupus rash to flare and may even trigger a serious flare of the disease itself. When outdoors on a sunny day, wear protective clothing (long sleeves, a big-brimmed hat), and use lots of sunscreen.
- If you are a young woman with lupus and wish to have a baby, work closely with your healthcare team to find the best treatment plan for you.

One main objective of *Fighting Lupus Battles: Living, Hoping, Searching, Climbing, Researching for the Cure* is for readers to hear from those who have to deal with lupus on a daily basis. Read about journeys of more lupus warriors in this section.

Gentle Hugs and Hope
"BB"

IT'S DARK AND raining, and I'm in pain. While I would like to crawl back into bed and forget the day and forget the pain, I have to rise because I have people who are depending on me today. This is my life with lupus every day.

It's hard not to flip flop all over the place when you're trying to put your words on paper, and it's even harder when you have brain fog.[1] It has been rather bad lately but I laugh, and so do those around me. If you don't keep your sense of humor, you're in for a world of hurt and frustration.

My journey really began around 1987, long before being diagnosed, when I was having my period for up to 23 days a month, with cramps so severe that I couldn't move. After one miscarriage, several D and C (dilation and curettage)[2] procedures, and a change in gynecologists, I was diagnosed with endometriosis.[3]

The treatment plan that I followed for more than a year ended up being successful, and I was finally given the all clear to get pregnant. The pregnancy turned high-risk when I started dilating

---

1   George Tsokos, MD, in 2018's *The Expert Series* sponsored by the Lupus Foundation of America, defined lupus brain fog as very mild cognitive dysfunction or impairment where things seem cloudy or heavily overcast. He further stated that many people with lupus express feelings of confusion, memory loss, and difficulty expressing their thoughts – overall slower cognitive function.

2   Curettage and dilation is a procedure to scrape and collect the tissue (endometrium) from inside the uterus. (Medline Plus)

3   Endometriosis is a disease in which the kind of tissue that normally grows inside the uterus grows outside the uterus. (Medline Plus)

and swelling at four and one-half months, so I was put on bedrest from the fifth month of pregnancy until delivery. It ended well in October of 1990 when our healthy 7 pound, 13 ounce baby became our second child. However, about one year later, I started having gynecological issues again and was advised to have a full hysterectomy[4]—not my choice.

In 1991, I started having debilitating back pain that affected my mobility, sometimes for days. I also experienced swelling and numbness in my legs, arms, and fingers. My mother's nurse suggested that I might have rheumatoid arthritis (RA).[5] I didn't know what that was, and I was sure I didn't have it. I forgot about his suggestion until my back went out again. My doctor ordered a magnetic resonance imaging (MRI).[6] After reviewing the results, my doctor referred me to a rheumatologist. I intended to follow up, but life and work got in the way.

The days and months went on until the numbness in my hands and pain in my arms became so bad that I would wake up screaming. I finally had to make a call, but it wasn't to a rheumatologist; it was to a neurosurgeon. The neurosurgeon ordered an electromyography (EMG).[7] With results and a safety pin in hand, the neuro said, "Can I see your hands?" Then he asked, "Are you dropping things? How long has this been going on?" All the while I was looking at that pin, wondering, *Where does he think he's going to stick that?* Then he asked me to turn my head.

Apparently he started sticking my fingers because he kept asking, "Can you feel that? Can you feel that?"

4	Hysterectomy is a surgery to remove a woman's uterus or womb. The uterus is the place where a baby grows when a woman is pregnant. (Medline Plus)

5	Rheumatoid arthritis, or RA, is a form of arthritis that causes pain, swelling, stiffness and loss of function in your joints." (MedlinePlus)

6	MRI uses a large magnet and radio waves to look at organs and structures inside the body. (MedlinePlus)

7	Electromyography (EMG) is a test that checks the health of the muscles (MedlinePlus).

Fighting Lupus Battles

I kept saying, "No."

I turned back to look at him, and each of my fingers had a speck of blood. I was scared at that point, not because of the blood but because I hadn't felt anything. Then he took that little hammer, you know the one that they use to test your reflexes in your knees, except he went for the elbow. I went through the roof.

"What the hell was that zap, and why did you do that?"

After I caught my breath, he said, "You have carpal tunnel syndrome in both hands and ulnar nerve damage in both elbows, and you need to see a rheumatologist after you have surgery."

Again that rheumatologist name popped up, but I wasn't thinking about that. I was thinking about having surgery in both arms. How? Why? When? Carpal tunnel release and ulnar nerve transposition surgeries for the right arm and hand were done on April 8, 2009. Then in September of 2009, I had ulnar nerve transposition surgery for my left arm.

All hell broke loose with my body in 2010. The fatigue arrived and hugged me so tight that breathing was almost impossible. The full body pain was so bad that I couldn't think or eat. I was certain that it had something to do with both surgeries I had the previous year, so I called the surgeon.

When I saw him, he asked, "Did you ever call that rheumatologist?"

Why does this keep popping up in conversations?

When I replied "No," he said, "Well you need to, and you need to fast. Better yet, I will call for you."

He left the room. Twenty minutes later, he returned and handed me a paper with a name, address and time for my appointment.

The day came in June 2010; you know, the one with that rheumatologist guy who kept popping up in conversations. During my visit, the doctor examined my joints, ordered laboratory tests, and had me arrange another appointment. Two weeks later, I saw him again.

I noticed that his face looked calm and soft as he took my hand in his and said, "How are you holding up?"

I was thinking, *Hold up, what does that mean?* But instead I said, "Oh, I'm fine."

He sat down and put on his glasses. I thought, *NO. Not the glasses, that's never a good sign.* He started flipping papers and marking them with his pen. Then he looked at me as the glasses came off. He proceeded to tell me that I have rheumatoid arthritis and, and, and, and…. I can't tell you anything else honestly because I could no longer hear what he was saying except for the words "chronic" and "no cure." I just stared at him. He wrote down something and handed it to me as he told me to research it. He also told me to get the prescription filled and make an appointment to see him again in two weeks.

I sat in my car sobbing. The doctor's rush of jumbled words flowed through my brain. The drive home was a blur. Once home, I started my Google search. The first word I searched was methotrexate, and I saw cancer, chemotherapy and DMARD (disease-modifying antirheumatic drugs). I sobbed some more. Do I have that? I can't remember what he said. The next drug I googled was Savella, used for nerve pain and depression. While I was all about help with the nerve pain, I wasn't depressed. Then came Cellcept, used to lower your body's immune system. When someone from the pharmacy called, I asked about those three drugs and started crying again right then and there. The script they filled was prednisone, a steroid used for treating inflammation.

At my next visit with the doctor, we decided I would take methotrexate, prednisone, and Savella and return in one month. I began taking the meds the next day. I started with 20mg of prednisone a day for 1 week, then 15mg, then 10mg, then steady on 5mg. These

Fighting Lupus Battles

were some of my thoughts: *Whoa, who am I, and what happened? I am sweating, hungry, angry, and emotional, plus sleeping a lot. What's that?* After my first injection of methotrexate, I had diarrhea. Plus I was puking, sweating, not eating, and sleeping most of the time. By the third day of taking Savella, I had a rash, with swollen eyes and lips. Plus the air hurt my skin, and tears burned my face. The doctor said, "Well, it's an allergic reaction to the Savella. Stop it and continue with the rest." Each Sunday was the same thing with the methotrexate: Monday was my sleep day; Tuesday was maybe eat day; Wednesday was stay close to the bathroom day; Thursday was better; and I was back to normal on Friday. Lowering the prednisone each week made living with me more tolerable.

The one-month return visit included an exam and blood work. Then came the phone call. "We have now added in Sjogren's syndrome. It's systemic, meaning it affects the entire body. So this time we're adding Plaquenil." What? Again, I went to the computer. Sjogren's syndrome is a disease in which the immune system attacks the glands that make tears and saliva, causing dry mouth and dry eyes. As the tears flowed, I could still see the words "chronic," "no cure."

After the third week of taking the Plaquenil, I started having vision issues. My eyesight was blurry, my peripheral vision was distorted, and my eyes felt like they were bouncing. The doctor lowered the dose. Next, diarrhea kicked in, and my hair started falling out. I was not a happy person. At month three, labs had not changed very much, so I was advised to add Humira, a TNF (tumor necrosis factor), for at least three to six months, while still taking methotrexate, prednisone and Plaquenil. So then I was injecting, swallowing, not eating, losing weight, losing hair, and feeling like life was passing by me.

For years after Humira, my doctors tried several other drugs that caused side effects or failed to work for me. I stopped injecting methotrexate after four and a half years. I stopped taking the

Gentle Hugs and Hope

Plaquenil because of vision issues, including the beginning of glaucoma in the right eye.

After years of having a good connection with my rheumatologist, I felt a change in him. I tried to continue with him, but I finally moved on to other rheumatologists until I found one who worked well with me. Finally, the Golden Ticket...sound the horns. He guided me, let me cry, and reassured me that he would do all he could to help me. And it was he who told me I have LUPUS. He told me that I had had it from the beginning, along with RA and Sjogren's. Imagine my shock!

In 2014, I suffered from back pain that was relieved through surgery. In 2015, I suffered with headaches, vision, and sinus problems and decided it was time to see the ENT (ear, nose, and throat specialist). Doctors discovered that I had two brain aneurysms that had to be fixed before surgery on my sinuses. They also announced that I had Raynaud's disease.

At that point, I felt defeated and alone. For the first time in seven years, I could no longer pretend that I wasn't a little depressed. I took off the mask and started meeting with a therapist monthly. It was a great help to just let it all out and begin a new freedom. It was the best present I could ever have given myself. I am currently taking prednisone, and the dosage varies between 10mg to 15mg daily. I am also receiving treatment in a pain clinic.

I have learned that lupus is not just a "ME" disease, it's a "WE" disease—spouse, partner, significant other, children, and friends. It affects every relationship that we have. I am thankful my husband is still here with me. I'm thankful he's my wingman, and I am thankful for his love. I also thank God for my support groups. I know that at any given time, I can get on the computer, and someone is there to walk me through, hold my hand, and let me know that I am not alone. We share the good, the bad, and the ugly. We also share the joys of marriage, children, grandchildren, graduations, and so much more. The bonds we have are like no other, and I am eternally grateful for them. We are more than just our diseases; we are family.

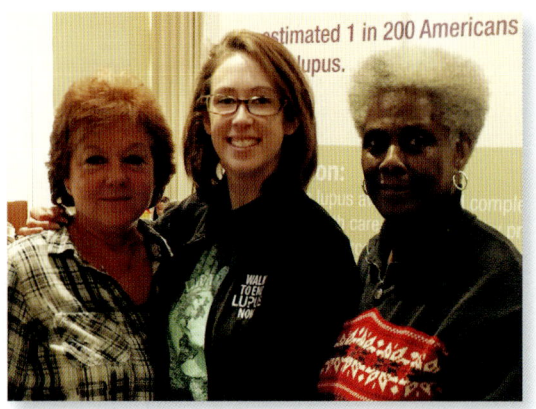

"BB" (left) with Sarah Spadoni and Kay Mimms

Commentary by Dr. Rosalind Ramsey-Goldman

Medication side effects are sometimes more troubling than the symptoms from the disease. In addition, it is very hard to live with a chronic illness that affects all parts of your life including family, friends, and co-workers. Working with your doctor to personalize your medication plan and minimize side effects is key. It is helpful to talk with a therapist, especially if you are in pain, depressed, or anxious as you deal with lupus. Research is one of the ways to help find new treatments, and both patients and doctors need to work together on this important mission. Participating in research can be a scary idea, but learning more about the different kinds of research, talking to someone who has participated in research, and understanding the consenting process which includes protections for the person who does research will help you learn about research and how it is done..

The Newest Addition to the Branch Family

Duwana Branch

So, you want to know about my ongoing journey with this thing called lupus, the newest addition to the Branch family? Shoot, I want to know myself. Normally, we experience joy and excitement when there is an addition being born into the family. On one hand, the lupus addition made me feel downright miserable and upset because I had no idea why my body and my health seemed to be failing. On the other hand, I was relieved to learn there was finally a name I could put to what I was living through.

My story began with me growing up as an asthmatic child. I was in and out of the hospital a lot, and that was by no means fun. That was the beginning of my hate/hate relationship with hospitals and needles. In my preteen years, my monthly cycles were so horrific that birth control pills were prescribed to regulate them. My appendix had to be removed in my senior year of high school. After the surgery, I started experiencing leg twitches and insomnia. At age twenty-two, I caught pneumonia and ended up in the hospital with a collapsed lung. When I was 28 years old, large gallstones developed, and I had my gallbladder removed. Ten days before my 30th birthday, my daughter was delivered early because I started to develop preeclampsia (high blood pressure and protein in my urine).

Things seemed to start spiraling down hill in 2010. I felt exhausted all the time. I experienced dizziness and excessive edema (swelling) in my hands, legs, and feet. I politely took myself to my primary care physician to see what was going on. Lab results and monitoring revealed that my vitamin D level was low, that I had high blood pressure, and that I was very close to being a diabetic. My doctor prescribed blood pressure medication. She also recommended that I follow a low-salt and low-carbohydrate diet and take an over-the-counter vitamin D supplement.

During the summer of 2012, I experienced unexplained excessive hair loss, and I was having extreme pain during my menstrual cycle. It was so bad that I thought I might be going through "the change." I could not walk, stand, or sit for very long. I could barely walk up the one five-step flight of stairs in my house. After about one year of trying to deal with those issues, I finally had an ultrasound that revealed a cyst on each of my ovaries. My obstetrics and gynecology (ob/gyn) doctor, who specialized in the health of the female reproductive system, recommended exploratory surgery. The plan was to remove the cysts first and then to explore the uterus. They discovered two conditions. One was endometriosis, or endo, and the second was adenomyosis. I knew about endo because many of my family members suffered through that condition and ended up having a hysterectomy. I was thinking, *I know about the endo. But what the hell is adenomyosis?* The ob/gyn explained it as a condition of the uterus where the cells that normally form a lining on the inside of the uterus also grow in the muscle wall of the uterus. He went on to explain that it could be caused by cells invading the muscle from prior surgery or by the lining tissue being deposited on the uterine muscle while I was pregnant. I realized another possibility as I read my doctor's notes. They suggested that inflammation of the uterine lining after the birth of my daughter could have caused cells to pass into the weakened muscle layer. So, on May 15, 2013, I had a partial hysterectomy.

After a month or so of recuperating, I felt ninety percent better. I still felt exhausted and tired often, but I chalked it up to the healing process. So in late June of the same year, I went back to work feel-

The Newest Addition to the Branch Family

ing pretty good. One day as I was walking from the train to my job, I noticed itchy red spots on my hands and arms. When I arrived at work, one of my co-workers asked me why I had red patches on my face. I didn't know where the patches came from, but I knew I was itching like crazy. After a couple of hours, the itching and red patches went away. This continued until the end of October or so. By that time, I wasn't sleeping well. When I managed to fall asleep, I was jolted awake by shooting pains everywhere. My joints hurt all the time, and it was becoming increasingly hard to walk and climb stairs again. I had no idea what was going on. I think what took the cake for me was not being able to write or pick things up without hurting. Working was becoming increasingly difficult.

In February 2014, my primary care physician, after completing comprehensive lab work and monitoring, gave me my dreaded diagnosis. I will never forget it. I was sitting at my desk at work when my doctor called. She told me that I had diabetes, high blood pressure, high cholesterol, peripheral neuropathy, and lupus. She gave me a brief description of lupus and told me to pick up my medication for everything except the lupus. To have my lupus monitored, she referred me to a rheumatologist. Then there was silence. Our phones disconnected. After sitting in my chair for about 15 minutes, I slowly got up out of the chair, gathered my things, told my boss I wasn't feeling well, and left the office. I think I sat in my car crying for about 20 minutes. I don't quite remember anything else about that day. The next day I called the rheumatologist and scheduled an appointment for the following month.

After three weeks of relying only on Google searches for information, my appointment date arrived. My husband went with me for this first appointment. We were led to an exam room.

The doctor came in and asked, "What brings you in today?"

Fighting Lupus Battles

I verbally gave him the rundown of all my issues as well as my lab results.

After my whole spiel, this man came back with, "Are you depressed because you have a lot of issues going on?"

Then he turns to my husband and says, "What do you think, sir?"

The doctor was talking to my husband, not me.

So my husband chimed in, "Well, I think she does suffer from depression. It doesn't make sense why there are so many varying issues."

My heart sank to the bottom of my stomach. I couldn't believe it.

I politely told both of them, "I am not depressed. I'm frustrated because I don't know why I am having these issues."

Then the doctor suggested that I might not have lupus, that I may have some other autoimmune issue.

He added, "Only time will tell".

He did a physical exam where he noted stiffness and such. That was it. He said that he would prescribe an anti-psychotic to help me cope, but I told him no, because I wasn't depressed. He asked me to go get some labs done and to make a follow-up in a month to go over the more comprehensive labs. I left that office feeling like no one heard me; I felt defeated.

I saw a new rheumatologist again in May of 2014. My lab results showed inflammation, and the rheumatologist saw that my joints were inflamed and swollen, so he prescribed prednisone and Plaquenil. In June of the same year, I went back for a medication follow-up and was too outdone by the fact that he didn't read my chart before he came into the room. I understand that doctors see a lot of patients, but at the same time, we patients want to be treated as if doctors give a damn about the people who come to

The Newest Addition to the Branch Family

see them, not as if we are some number like jail inmates. So that was the last time I saw that guy.

My next rheumatologist and I got along great. He took my labs and reviewed records from my other doctors—primary care, dermatologist, hematologist, and previous rheumatologist. I'd say my first appointment with him was awesome. It lasted for about an hour. He was very detailed about the process of narrowing down my symptoms. He also informed me that my symptoms would come and go as well as change. Our relationship was great.

Unfortunately, in January 2016, my husband's job changed insurance carriers. The new carrier had a different provider network. How did that affect me? I had to move on from my primary care and my newfound and great rheumatologist because they were not in our new provider network. So now what? I had no rheumatologist, no primary care physician, and no medication refills, but I still had lots of pain, swelling, high blood pressure and diabetic issues. I was really down and out. I started to withdraw again. Joining a support group and attending meetings helped me cope.

Nine months later, in September, I finally found a new primary care doctor. She started helping me to get my diabetes and blood pressure in check. She was also able to refer me to a rheumatologist who was a part of our network. I could see the new rheumatologist the following month.

In October when I saw my new rheumatologist, I was happy to hear that she knew my previous rheumatologist. My new rheumy was just as inviting as my last one. Like with previous doctors, the relationship with the new rheumatologist got off to a rocky start at first. It took about six months to get us on track. Now, I am able to ask questions without feeling like I'm not being heard. We have a true dialogue about all my ailments. It's very refreshing.

The additions to the Branch family are currently high blood pressure, high cholesterol, diabetes, lupus, Raynaud's disease,

Fighting Lupus Battles

glaucoma, autoimmune urticaria (hives), and polyneuropathy. Wow, that's quite a mouthful. Now I receive care and treatments from my rheumatologist, dermatologist, ophthalmologist and primary care physician. I am taking twelve different medications that consist of about 18 pills per day, plus four puffs of asthma medication. It has been a rough journey getting to a headspace that has allowed me to be somewhat ok with my health issues. Each day seems like a long winding road that needs to be navigated with precision for me to get through it. My journey has been filled with ups and downs, letdowns, and disappointments from people who are supposed to love you unconditionally. Why is it that in a time of great peril and confusion people pull away from you?

I finally have some answers to the painstaking question of what is going on with me, but it still doesn't answer my question of why. I hope that as time goes on in my quest, I will get to the end of the rainbow. I also hope that my story will help anyone dealing with any autoimmune issues. I want to thank my family for helping to give me the courage to keep fighting.

Commentary by Dr. Rosalind Ramsey-Goldman

I do not think that I could have said this any clearer: Being diagnosed with lupus is like getting a new member of the family. It affects everything about you. Support from family and friends is a key part of dealing with the unknowns of lupus, which change day to day, sometimes even minute to minute. It is important to find a healthcare provider who you trust. Unfortunately, other circumstances, like changes in insurance, can interfere with those relationships. Healthcare providers can also be impacted by those external factors since we help patients with chronic illnesses. We also feel a sense of loss when our patients have to switch to another clinic.

Lupus Survivor and Advocate: I'm Blessed

Patricia A. Brumley

IN 1990, I started feeling tired all the time, and I just didn't know what was going on. I was also suffering from joint pain and having problems with my feet. I ended up having surgery on my left foot that year. Then the next year, I had surgery on my right foot.

In 1993, I decided that I wanted to have a child. I was two and a half months into my pregnancy when I lost the baby. I ended up having to have a partial hysterectomy, also called subtotal or supracervical hysterectomy where just the upper part of the uterus is removed. (US Department of Health and Human Services—Office of Women's Health). After having the surgery, I became very depressed and could not understand why all those things were happening to me. I continued to have a lot of joint pain, but no doctor was able to tell me why. So I just went back and forth seeing doctors and taking all kinds of tests, trying to see what the problem was. Being in so much pain caused me to miss many days at work.

In early 1996, I noticed I was getting bald spots on my head, and I was exhausted all the time, so I decided to see a dermatologist. During the visit, I could tell that the doctor knew what was wrong, but she refused to say until she did a biopsy. A week later, I was called into her office where I was given the diagnosis: discoid lupus. I had no idea what lupus was, and so the first thing I asked the doctor was, "Am I going to die?" Of course, she said no, and she sat me down for a long talk. My best friend, Karon, was with me for both visits with the dermatologist.

Fighting Lupus Battles

Later, I went to see a rheumatologist. After taking test after test, I was diagnosed with systemic lupus erythematosus—lupus. At that time, I was still scared to death, but I was beginning to understand why I was always in pain and exhausted all the time.

After getting over the shock, I knew I had to make sure I kept all of my doctor appointments even though I was still teaching. I also had to follow the doctors' orders. I discovered that I needed to learn all I could about this crazy disease. At times, I stayed to myself because I didn't want to be around my family or anyone. My family members were having a hard time understanding what I was going through. So I started sharing lupus information with them, hoping it would help them to understand why I acted the way I did at times. It took some time, but my family was there for me. When I had doctors' appointments either my sister, Anita, or Karon would take off work to be with me. I thank God for my family and my best friend.

Later, I met Annette Peete, who had been diagnosed with lupus years before we met. She took me under her wing and helped me through that scary period of my life. Toward the end of 1996, Annette asked if I would be interested in starting a lupus support group, and I said yes. We both recognized the need for a comprehensive approach to empowering individuals who deal with lupus. Lupus patients need empowerment in order to pursue productive, independent and fulfilling lives. I became co-founder of the Life with Lupus Guild. We held meetings on the first Saturday of each month at Chicago's Apostolic Church of God under the late Bishop Arthur M. Brazier. I made up my mind that no matter what, I will be an advocate for lupus until God calls me home.

I lost my friend Annette Peete in March of 2006 after her long battle with lupus. I said to myself, *I will do whatever I have to do to keep Annette's dream alive.* Later I reconstructed the Lupus Guild and renamed it "Living Life" with Lupus Support Group. Bettie Carter and Wanda Dowdell became board members.

Lupus Survivor and Advocate: I'm Blessed

I thank God for having a supportive family because without them, I don't think I would have made it this far. I had to depend on them for so much, especially after having a left knee replacement in 1999, right knee replacement in 2006, another left knee replacement in 2014, and so many other health challenges. As my father would always say, "Family must stick together no matter what, because without family you have nothing."

Through all of my trials and tribulations I have become a wiser and stronger person. I thank God every day for being the head of my life.

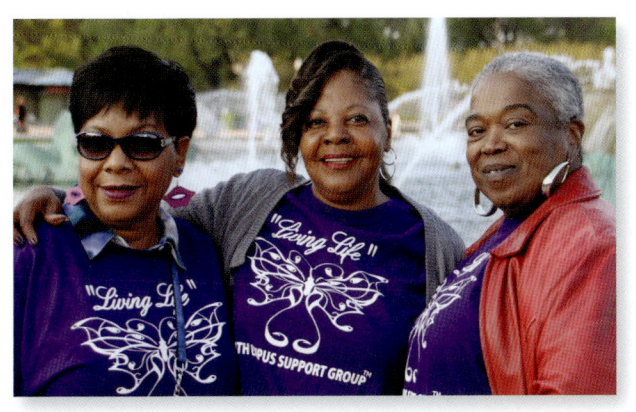

Wanda Dowdell, Bettie Carter, and Pat Brumley

Commentary by Dr. Rosalind Ramsey-Goldman
Taking charge of your health is empowering. Teaching and sharing knowledge is a strategy for empowerment when you feel lost. Supporting others and getting support for self is a recurrent theme of lupus warriors.

Name that Disease: What is Lupus?

Bettie Carter

MOVING TO CALIFORNIA after having my first child at age seventeen brought promises of big things and warmer weather. I was looking forward to living in a big-time state that didn't have the cold and snow like in Chicago. So I boarded a Greyhound bus, looking forward to getting married, adopting my future husband's daughter from another relationship, and creating a new life in California.

While living in California for the next four years, I felt like I was living the life. We got married, and I held several jobs—procurement clerk, assistant buyer, and buyer. Then we had another daughter and moved to Virginia, where we had our fourth daughter. At that point, we were a big happy family with four girls—Tamara, Tabitha, Teri and Tisha. I hadn't finished high school, so I took night classes to earn my high school diploma while I also worked part-time. Even though life was stressful raising four young children, going to school, and working, I was still able to maintain good health. The only health problem I had during that time was a minor cold.

We moved to Chicago for a couple of years. Then in 1985, we moved back to California. This time I wanted to get my body in shape because I was thinking of becoming a centerfold girl for Jet Magazine. I had the looks and just needed to tone my body. I worked out in the gym three days a week, ran five miles two days a week, and rode my bike a few miles. Well, my plan didn't work; Jet Magazine turned me down, but it was worth the effort. I continued working out for a couple of years because I wanted to

Name that Disease: What is Lupus?

keep my nice shape. I also met my friend, Carolyn, who is like a sister to me.

After my husband and I divorced in 1993 and my mother became very ill in 1994, I decided to return to Chicago. Having hitched my 1988 Ford station wagon to the back of a U-Haul truck, my sister and I drove to Chicago with my two youngest daughters. We drove for two days non-stop, through two rainstorms, while suffering from sleep deprivation and fatigue.

I appreciate my sister, Ludella, for letting me and my daughters stay with her while I searched for a job. I finally found one at a warehouse where they made car interior parts like door handles, window locks, and radio knobs. The smell of wax and metal was in the air from all the melting of different materials. After working there for three weeks, I became sick. I was suffering from light-headedness, swollen hands and eyes, and redness in my face. I quit the job and started going to doctors. I went to the emergency room at least three times within two weeks. They did a visual exam and gave me cream for everything. So, I was thinking, *OK, my body is trying to adjust to the Midwest weather; plus that long road trip is starting to have an effect on me.*

After about three months of going back and forth to doctors, I felt better, so I began another job search. In February 1995, I started working at Marshall Field's in downtown Chicago. I said, "Thank you, Jesus." I was working there for only about a month before I started getting sick all over again. I was thinking, *This can't be happening to me. I am a very healthy lady, 35 years young. My body is just trying to adjust to the change in climate.* I went to a health clinic and was determined to stay until somebody told me what was wrong with me. I had to wait for five hours before I saw a doctor. After spending only ten minutes with me, the doctor diagnosed a bad cold or rash, gave me more cream, and sent me home without doing any type of tests. I was very disappointed. I started taking all kinds of over-the-counter cold medicine. Something

Fighting Lupus Battles

must have worked because I started to feel better, so I began searching for another job.

On March 4, 1995, I went to bed around 11 p.m. I got up about 1 or 2 a.m. to use the bathroom. The next thing I knew I woke up in the ER. I was cold and confused. When a nurse came in to give me a blanket, I asked her what happened.

She said, "Oh you passed out and have lupus; you will be all right." I was thinking, *Lupus? What's that?*

Then I asked her, "What is lupus?"

"Oh", she said, "you haven't seen the doctor yet?"

I answered, "No."

Then she said, "He will tell you what to do."

As she left the room, I turned my head to the wall, and tears rolled down my face. My first thought was, *I'm going to die.* Then, I thought, *What am I going to tell my family?* They all know I've been sick, but they don't know what's wrong with me. All I know is that they took blood from me while I was unconscious, and that's it.

The doctor came in and said, "You have lupus, which is a disease". He talked to me for a brief minute about lupus, gave me another doctor's name, and told me to go see him. Then he gave me some pain pills and more cream—yes, more cream. All the time I was still thinking about what the doctor meant when he said, "You have lupus, which is a disease." It's a disease….Really?

On my way home, I was in shock. I didn't say anything to my family or my friend because I needed more information. Once I had a little strength and before going to see the new doctor, I tried to find information about lupus at the library. The only thing I found was a book about a wolf. A doctor wrote the book; I wanted something from a person who had been diagnosed with lupus. The Internet had a lot of information about the immune system, but there was

Name that Disease: What is Lupus?

nothing that I could put my finger on about lupus. I didn't know what I could do to get information about lupus.

I went to see the new doctor—a rheumatologist. He was very patient with me. He listened to my every word and allowed me to talk to him as long as I needed. I thank God for him because I feel in my soul that he was a good doctor who saved my life. It took a while, but the Plaquenil and steroids that he prescribed started working. Then two months after being on those meds, I started experiencing symptoms again—pain, swollen feet and hands, and redness in my face and eyes. It was very depressing. I didn't want my kids to see me cry, so I would stay in the bathtub for long periods of time. When the kids checked on me, I would throw water on my face so they wouldn't see the tears. That went on for about four months before the doctor tried another medicine, methotrexate.

Now, the methotrexate had a lot of side effects, but the doctor told me it was the best thing he could give me since the Plaquenil didn't work for me. I started out on 40mg of prednisone and 15mg of methotrexate. I weighed 116 pounds all my life, but after I started the new regiment of prednisone and methotrexate, I gained 35 pounds. I didn't care, though, because I started to feel a lot better.

My family saw that I was sick all the time. Some days I couldn't even get out of bed. So I decided to tell my kids and family about my lupus diagnosis. At first, they thought lupus was cancer and that I was going to die. Later, they started taking it better than I thought they would. Sometimes, we could even joke about my condition. I remember when my daughter graduated from 8th grade. We didn't have a car and had to walk four blocks to the church where the graduation was to be held. My feet were swollen to the point that I had to wear house shoes.

My daughter Teri said, "Mom, you don't have to come."

Fighting Lupus Battles

I told her, "I will be there—me and my big elephant feet." We laughed so hard.

By August 1995, I was feeling like I could climb Mount Everest. I had a lot of energy, and my body was not in pain. I had no swelling and no redness in my face or eyes. My oldest daughter was due to have her baby in September, and I felt like I could go back to work. The same day I had a job interview at Carson's downtown was the same day she went into labor. I thought, *Oh my goodness, what am I going to do?* Tabitha reminded me that I had wanted to work for a long time, and she insisted that I complete the interview. I got the job, and she had my first granddaughter—Tatiana.

For two years while working at Carson's, I was doing well—only having a few flare-ups here and there. When I had a flare, I would go to the ER where I was given steroids and an injection of morphine. Then things would get back to normal for a while. I knew the steroids could affect my bones, but I didn't think it would be such a rapid process. I started having problems with my bones. First, I had to have a total hip replacement. I was thinking, *I am too young for this, and what will I look like with an artificial hip?* Less than two years later, I had to have my other hip replaced. Later I had to have my left shoulder replaced. Then my knees started giving me problems, not bad enough to have them replaced, but I did get shots in them for a couple of years. The cane became part of my wardrobe. I was really confused and started thinking, *I can't work because my bones are not good.*

I continued to have problems with my bones in different parts of my body. I had surgery on my feet. My teeth, which had always been healthy, started just falling out of my mouth. Getting false teeth was a very, very hard decision for me. I could live with having hip and shoulder replacements because people can't see the scars. But my mouth and my smile can be seen; plus having an upper partial was a weird feeling to get used to. But I still looked good. In fact, nobody knew I had false teeth until now.

Name that Disease: What is Lupus?

In 2006, I took a flight from Chicago to California to see my girlfriend, Carolyn, and I sat during the entire flight. I made it to Carolyn's house, but within two hours, I couldn't walk or stand up straight. I was rushed by ambulance to a medical facility where they diagnosed me with sciatica.[1] After returning home and seeing my doctor, I had to have back surgery.

Also in 2006, I started having heart palpitations. I was required to wear a heart monitor off and on for seven years. The results showed nothing was amiss until the last heart monitor test. In December 2015, I had an echo Doppler on my heart, and it was explained to me that I have an enlarged aorta.

This has been a long road for me since I was diagnosed with systemic lupus. I have had hip replacements (one replacement done a second time; the other needing to be redone), a shoulder replacement, knees that need injections, surgically repaired feet, false teeth, surgically repaired back, a tube in my right ear, enlarged aorta, and sciatica. However, I never had a bad flare where I had to stay in the hospital overnight. I must say, God has really blessed me.

My baby girl, Tisha, was also diagnosed with lupus. Her symptoms included aches, pain, and hair loss. Then two years later my aunt was diagnosed with systemic lupus, and she is having a lot of problems. Now I am thinking it has to be hereditary, and I suspect it's from my grandmother's side of the family.

I decided to join the "Living Life" Lupus Support Group. That support group saved my life. I was a very quiet person, and I didn't talk much. You couldn't pay me to speak to anybody about anything, especially to groups about me or my disease. But after joining the support group and hearing how the people who have lupus were not getting help, I felt that I needed to do something about it. It took me some

---

1   Sciatica is pain affecting the large nerve extending from the lower back down the back of each leg (MedlinePlus).

Fighting Lupus Battles

years to really speak up about lupus, but I thank God daily for giving me the voice.

I have been in remission for over ten years. During eight of those years, I've been involved in lupus advocacy, education, and research. I have spoken in Washington, DC to our congresswomen about more funding for lupus research. I have spoken about lupus at many events and through many avenues—radio, television, newspapers, schools, hospitals, health fairs, and the 97th Illinois General Assembly. I have traveled to Detroit, Michigan, and Milwaukee, Wisconsin, to support their lupus fundraisers as well as to make donations to other lupus organizations. I am an advocate for lupus, and it really makes me feel amazing. I have done lupus walks and lupus studies. I manage three lupus pages on Facebook, trying to help people all over the world. I have met some beautiful people in these 22 years as a lupus survivor and warrior. Sometimes we talk on the phone for hours, just so I can be that ear for someone who needs to be heard. As crazy as it may sound, I don't think I would change anything because God gave me this gift to help others. It feels wonderful to be able to be there for them.

When I was first diagnosed and spoke to people, they would always ask, "What is lupus? I know somebody who died from lupus." Now they say, "Oh, I know about lupus; my sister and my friend have it, and they are doing good." That indicates to me that we have made progress in spreading the word about lupus. We have come a long, long way toward increasing lupus awareness. That makes me feel good, but we still have a long way to go.

I will keep fighting to bring more awareness to lupus, to help lupus survivors live a better life, and to help find a cure. I believe God is keeping me as healthy as I am so I can keep helping other people.

Name that Disease: What is Lupus?

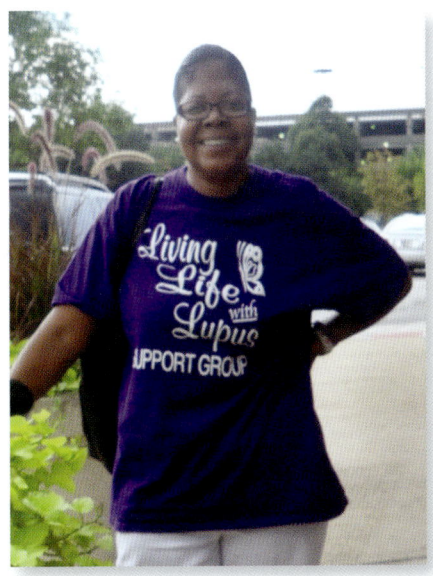

Bettie Carter

Commentary by Dr. Rosalind Ramsey-Goldman

There is no known cause of lupus. The question of genetics is frequently asked when a person is diagnosed with lupus. When one thinks about a genetic disease, examples that come to mind are sickle cell disease or cystic fibrosis. In those two conditions, there is one gene that is not working properly or is missing, leading to the medical problems. In lupus, there may be many genes, even up to 100, contributing to the risk, but genetics is probably not enough to explain the cause of the disease. Factors in the environment also play a role and may impact how genes work. Finding the responsible gene(s) and the environmental triggers is a focus of many research studies.

Lupus: My Beginnings, No End

Donna L. Emery

THANK GOD FOR family. In my early childhood, everything was everything with my family. I am the oldest of four girls. I was always a hard worker. I never complained about anything until I started being sick with colds and chills all the time. My mom took me to the doctor, who said I was anemic. He said that I needed to take some large dark pills to help my anemia. I think that was the beginning of my battles with lupus.

Next came my heavy menstrual periods, pains, and headaches, with bleeding forever, sometimes for weeks. The doctor mentioned that I should take birth control pills, but my mom was not having that. The doctor also mentioned something about my red and white blood cells. But he said it was nothing for my mom to worry about. I learned how to deal with all those challenges as best I could, one way or another.

During my first marriage, I realized I had a serious problem. I was very sick—fainting and very depressed. I had no clue as to what was happening. After having a baby born with Down syndrome, I wondered, *What is wrong with me?* But, you learn how to survive. My beautiful daughter, Deanna, was only eight months old when she passed away, yet I continued to push through everything to survive.

By the 1990s when I was in my forties, I was married again and trying to live a happy life. I was enjoying my family and career, but my illness continued to change everything. I felt like I was losing my mind. Hoping to find out what was going on with me, my ex-hus-

Lupus: My Beginnings, No End

band encouraged me to see his physician. She ran various blood tests to find out if I had lupus. She was correct. She diagnosed me with systemic lupus erythematosus (SLE). For many years, I wanted to know what was going on with me. Finally one doctor ran the various tests, and now I know. She saved my life.

What is lupus? Lupus is an illness that changed my entire life forever. Throughout my life, I dealt with fatigue, achiness, stiffness, fever, swollen glands, stress, hair loss, sleeplessness, and pain in my fingers and hands—everything hurting. My new doctor recommended that I see a rheumatologist. What a doctor! We connected the very first visit as he helped me to understand what was going on in my body. I thought I was crazy with this illness, but he helped me to understand everything—the hair loss, chills, headaches, sweats, and never sleeping. I experienced a big challenge in 2011 when I had open-heart bypass surgery.[1] I survived. Thank you, God!

Every three to four months, I see my rheumatologist for lupus monitoring and blood tests. The blood tests include antinuclear antibody (ANA), complement C3, creatinine, urinalysis, comprehensive metabolic panel, hemoglobin a1c, lipid panel, thyroid stimulating hormone (TSH), and complete blood count (CBC). I don't have a problem having to do all the blood tests because it makes me feel like I'm ahead of the game. To me, having to do all the blood tests just means that I am here another day to live and fight all the way.

I thank God for many things He has allowed me to experience. In 2018, I retired from Young & Rubicam Chicago Advertising after 39 years as a broadcast traffic manager. Thank God for my job and for all the people who supported me through all my ups and down with lupus. I thank God for my family: my mom, my sisters, my daughter Maya, and my grandchildren, Olivia and Noah. I also thank Him for my best girlfriends, Alfreda and Yvetta, for the

---

1   Bypass is a surgery in which a healthy artery or vein is connected to a blocked heart artery (MedlinePlus).

Fighting Lupus Battles

South Suburban Hospital Lupus Support Group, and of course for my ex-husband who helped me through the challenges and all the pain.

Being a survivor is what lupus warriors are today. Donna Emery is a lupus survivor. I am a lupie!

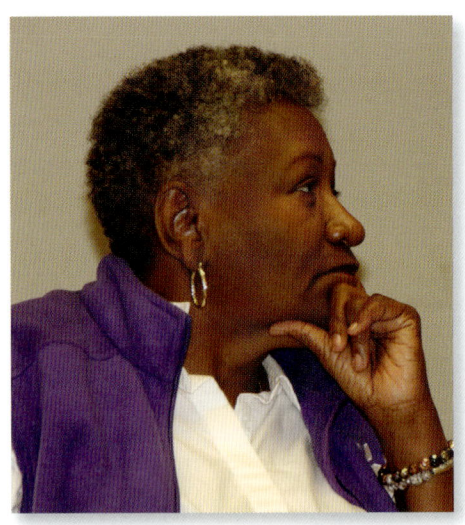

Donna Emery

Commentary by Dr. Rosalind Ramsey-Goldman
There are recurrent themes expressed in the stories shared in this book, including symptoms that come and go, unremitting fatigue, knowing you are not feeling right but no one knows what is wrong with you, strains on personal relationships, and depression during the long journey to diagnosis. Finding a healthcare provider you trust, finding medications that work for you, and having support systems summarize the basis of the success of how these lupus warriors cope with their disease.

Finding Understanding, Hoping for a Cure

Chris Fragassi

THE FIRST TIME I remember hearing of lupus was in the 1989 movie *Gross Anatomy*, in which the character played by Christine Lahti has lupus. In the movie, she is a doctor who orders a medical student to diagnose a complex illness. He accurately completes the assignment, not knowing that it is her illness of lupus that he has diagnosed. I didn't know anything about lupus then, but it was clear from the movie that it was a puzzling disease that was difficult to diagnose and seemed to be a medical mystery. I didn't really think about it again until the early 1990s when I saw a doctor for an apparent allergy to penicillin. I was breaking out in hives, and my hands were swelling up. When the doctor looked at my hands, he noticed that I had rashes on the palms of my hands. He asked me if anyone ever mentioned lupus to me. At the time, I thought the doctor was exaggerating what to me was a simple allergic reaction, so I brushed it off. I thought about it again when it was clear that my chronic health issues were more than just allergies or chronic fatigue.

My struggles with lupus actually started when I was very young, before I had ever heard of lupus. I was often sick as a child with the usual childhood illnesses. I also experienced less common ones, like a kidney infection when I was 6, and chronic knee pain that started around the age of 12. The explanations that doctors gave for the knee pain varied from "growing pains," to being overweight, to "psychosomatic illness." The suggestion that these and other symptoms that I would later experience were "all in my head" caused me to even question the eventual diagnosis of lupus. For

Fighting Lupus Battles

years, I wondered if I really was just a hypochondriac, especially when I would experience bouts of good health or when doctors would give me a reasonable explanation for my puzzling symptoms, usually telling me it was "some sort of virus" or allergies.

It took years of consulting several doctors and countless diagnostic tests before I was diagnosed with lupus. Because I did have allergies, a lot of my strange symptoms were thought to be allergic in nature. My allergist was puzzled when I didn't respond to the treatments he prescribed. He thought I might have chronic fatigue syndrome, which was a common diagnosis back in the 1990s when a patient presented with severe fatigue. I was also told I might be depressed or just stressed, which might explain my severe fatigue. The laundry list of possible diseases even included lymphoma or leukemia. These were quickly ruled out, but the possibility that I might have these serious diseases frightened me.

The years of not knowing what was wrong with me but knowing that there was something wrong were frightening, confusing, and exhausting. The puzzling symptoms I experienced included pleurisy[1] and pericarditis.[2] Other puzzling symptoms were frequent flu-like illnesses, extreme fatigue and weakness, loss of appetite and subsequent 40-pound weight loss, headaches, lightheadedness, loss of balance, anxiety and panic attacks, and depression. The bouts of extreme fatigue and lightheadedness as well as panic attacks forced me to stop driving in my forties. That caused me to be depressed over the loss of my independence.

I was often judged and criticized for my frequent absences at work, and I worried constantly that I would lose my job. I became obsessed with finding out what was wrong with me. That obsession made some people think I was a hypochondriac because I

---

1   Pleurisy is an inflammation of the lining of the lungs and chest (the pleura) that leads to chest pain when you take a breath or cough.

2   Pericarditis is a condition in which the sac-like covering around the heart (pericardium) becomes inflamed (Medline Plus).

Finding Understanding, Hoping for a Cure

was so focused on my symptoms. I was fortunate that my two sisters also had similar symptoms. Although we all were frustrated that no doctors seemed to know what was causing our vague and puzzling symptoms, at least we had each other for support. As it turned out, we all have been diagnosed with lupus and fibromyalgia. My younger sister was the first one of us to be diagnosed with lupus. She had experienced many of the puzzling symptoms that I had and spent many years going from doctor to doctor until she finally got the diagnosis of lupus. It was her diagnosis that brought me to the rheumatologist who eventually diagnosed me with fibromyalgia and lupus. I was not surprised when I got the diagnosis. I was actually relieved that I finally had an answer to my strange symptoms. As much as having lupus scared me, at least I knew what I was dealing with.

Eventually my older sister was also diagnosed with lupus and fibromyalgia. She had also experienced years of appointments with doctors and countless diagnostic tests in the pursuit of getting answers to her puzzling symptoms. My two children also have been diagnosed with fibromyalgia, Raynaud's disease, and Crohn's disease.[3] It has been distressing to watch my children struggling with autoimmune diseases and having to live with chronic health issues. I hate that they are going through what I went through, but at least the answers have come a bit sooner for them than for me. I have tried to be an example for them in the way I cope with my illness. I want them to know that although it is not easy to live with chronic illness, it is possible to have a full life and not be defined by a disease. I also want them and all who have to deal with chronic illness to know that they need to be kind to themselves, take good care of their health, and set their own goals. No one needs to live up to someone else's expectations, especially someone who doesn't understand what it's like to live with a chronic disease.

---

3   Crohn's disease is a condition that causes inflammation of the digestive system (MedlinePlus).

Fighting Lupus Battles

It was so emotionally healing to meet others who were struggling with lupus when I joined a support group sponsored by the Lupus Society of Illinois. There I found people who understood what I was going through. I have met the most inspirational, courageous, and beautiful souls at the support group meetings. It has also been rewarding for me to offer support to others who have been recently diagnosed with lupus. When I was asked to take over as facilitator of the group, I hesitated only because it's hard to commit to things when you don't know how you'll feel, and I hate to let anyone down. But I thought about it, and I realized that my fellow "lupies" would truly understand if there were times I could not make a meeting. So I agreed, and I've never regretted it. I believe so strongly in support groups because they help people deal with painful or frightening experiences in their lives. It is so healing to talk about something that most people wouldn't understand. It helps to find understanding and support from people who are fighting the same battles. We share the hope that there will be new treatments and perhaps even a cure for lupus someday.

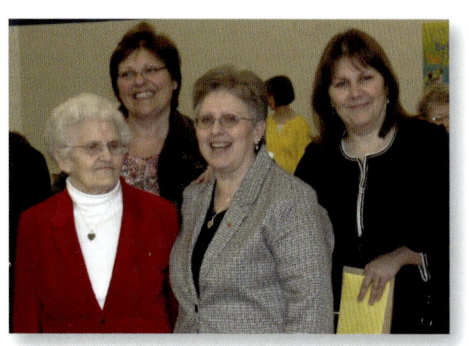

Chris Fragassi, right, with her mother and sisters

Commentary by Dr. Rosalind Ramsey-Goldman

Working can be challenging for those with lupus. You may look OK but feel terrible. You may feel fine one minute and then suddenly become very tired, have pain, or not be able to think clearly. Worrying about losing your job adds to the physical and emotional stress of having lupus. This is one of several stories describing trying to work despite lupus.

Lupus Testimony

Jasmine Henderson

I DON'T RECALL HOW much time we spent in my small dark hospital room. However, what I can recall quite clearly is lying on a stretcher, huddled and shivering in a mess of blankets, with the sound of my heartbeat pounding in my ears as I fall in and out of a vertigo-laden sleep. Periodically, I return to a semi-lucid state of consciousness, pleading for ice chips or vomiting black bile into the trash. My suffering, ceaseless and uncompromising, is given a name when the door to my room opens abruptly. I see a doctor's head peer in, his white beard leading his experienced face. The doctor's body never enters the room completely, giving his head a disembodied quality, as if it is operating independently of an actual body—a phantom haunting the hospital, dispensing sterile diagnoses to anxious patients, its brand of horror. The head speaks: "Looks like you have lupus, and your kidneys have failed." It disappears as quickly as it appeared, leaving a pronounced silence, with words and thoughts arrested in astonishment.

Hindsight, being what it is, reveals that my body has been expressing lupus symptoms since I was 18 years old. It began 17 years ago when I was a freshly independent college student. I tried my best to ignore my new recurring migraines and body aches, dismissing myself from class to step into the restroom to vomit, or occasionally missing class all together. I told myself my ailments were caused by the stresses of college life—the studying, the course load, and the late nights spent partying.

Fighting Lupus Battles

At 23, I recall being irritated by an odd feeling in my knees and shoulders, like I just couldn't get my joints to pop no matter how much I rotated them. Then I started to have a regular ache in my spine that I chalked up to the cheap college futon I was sleeping on. Even now I'm ashamed that it never occurred to me to see a doctor while I was still covered under my mother's insurance. It just didn't compute that in the prime of independence and youth, one could become sick and broken down for no apparent reason. It just made more sense to young adults to wish everything would work out. It infuriates me to this day to hear young people in their twenties accuse me of bringing this upon myself, by whatever means. It's probably a defense mechanism that keeps them from fearing for their own safety and livelihood.

By January 2005, I had graduated from college with my bachelor's degree and moved into a one-bedroom basement apartment with my boyfriend. One day I woke up to the noon sun flooding my bedroom. I attempted to roll over to shield my eyes from the light when a paralyzing pain sucked the breath from my body. It was like an electric shock permeating throughout my nervous system. Nothing wanted to move—not my arms, not my legs, not even my fingers. Fearfully, I called out to my boyfriend. Panicked, my boyfriend and I made plans to go to the emergency room. My boyfriend carefully began to dress me. He maneuvered my still body, manipulating my limbs into a hoodie and sweatpants. My joints loosened a bit, a small victory that didn't stop the tears from coursing down my face. I could barely raise my arms above my belly button on my own power.

Once I arrived at the hospital, the doctor on call said the results of my initial tests revealed I may have rheumatoid arthritis. She prescribed some prednisone, an anti-inflammatory, and some painkillers. She also gave me a referral to a rheumatologist. The reference was appreciated, but now that I was 25 years old, I was no longer covered by my parents' health insurance. I was em-

Lupus Testimony

ployed part-time at a retail job that paid $6.75 an hour. I was barely able to afford my rent and basic sustenance, let alone health insurance. I kept my appointment, but they turned me away at the receptionist desk. No insurance, no doctor.

The prednisone helped with the inflammation; I could move again. But I would inevitably run out of medicine, leaving me no recourse but to rack up more debt at the ER to get more, or, failing that, to self-medicate. This was my life. Every joint would swell. My knees were like doll heads. My knuckles were like King marbles, large and knotted. Unable to get in and out of bed without substantial pain, I resorted to sitting up in a living room chair to sleep. And for the love of God, don't let it rain. Most days, my boyfriend helped me dress. Even my jaws had become rigid. My boyfriend would prepare a meal of watered down oatmeal for me before dropping me off at work. Oatmeal and Ensure were the only things I could manage many days because I could sip them through a straw. My weight dropped from 115 pounds and danced between 90 and 105. Usually, I could get by on upping the dosage on over-the-counter arthritis meds, but every now and then the lining of my lungs would become inflamed as well. My breathing would become labored as pressure on my lungs seemed to increase. Then I was back in the ER for more prednisone. What an awful cycle!

One day in September 2005, while I was on a nice little cocktail of Advil and Vicodin, I felt well enough to get pregnant. I thought, *God has shined down and granted me a miracle.* Not only was I having a child, slowly but also surely, I was becoming like a normal person again. I could walk unencumbered by pain. I could yawn without wincing. I could even dance to the greatest hits of Whitney Houston. I ate huge breakfasts of whole milk, eggs, bacon, hash browns, and toast. Best of all, through the services of Planned Parenthood, I had health insurance! Since I was feeling better, I applied for and got a new job with better pay and company insurance as well. The preg-

Fighting Lupus Battles

nancy was going well. Occasionally, the doctors would mention some concern for my kidney function, but they assured me things would improve when the pregnancy was over. In June 2006, I gave birth to a beautiful, healthy baby girl!

Then one day in December 2006. I woke up to the sound of my alarm clock. My boyfriend rolled to his side of the bed in the dark. I had a splitting headache. My whole body felt sore. I really wanted to call off, but I had used my three sick days on some kind of mutant stomach flu. I proceeded with my morning routine. I showered, fed and dressed the baby, and packed the diaper bag for daycare. I ignored my swollen knees, the queasiness in my stomach, and the roaring of the blood in my ears. Finally I decided I absolutely had to do something about my increasing migraine. I went to find a muscle relaxer and ran into the wall. I backed away slowly thinking, *What the hell?* Suddenly it felt as if the floor had moved from under me, and I collapsed. I called to my boyfriend for help as the room spun around me. My boyfriend called his brother to keep an eye on our baby, and we headed once again to the hospital.

I was admitted and spent days of coming in and out of consciousness, with nurses coming and going and people explaining things that I couldn't hear or remember. I remember waking one evening to see a young doctor patiently sitting next to my bed. He quietly asked me how I was. Then he explained everything. I had been misdiagnosed with rheumatoid arthritis. I actually had lupus that must have gone into remission during my pregnancy, which was common. He said it was also common for the lupus to flare up after a pregnancy. Lupus had caused relentless damage to both kidneys. He said the stomach flu I had experienced was the beginning of the last stage of renal failure. He expressed his amazement that the rest of my organs were so intact. He told me I was very lucky.

Since then I've been on and off dialysis, have had two kidney transplants, and have not had a flare as severe as my two previous

Lupus Testimony

incidents. I continue to see the rheumatologist, take the immune suppressants prescribed, and try to live life like a "normal" person. That, I think, is the hardest part, redefining "normal." Normal is now a full schedule of doctor appointments and specialists. Normal is a collection of pills for breakfast, lunch and dinner. Normal is being acutely aware of my body—keeping track of my blood pressure and urine output, journaling aches and pains, and taking it seriously when I need rest. I've come to realize my body will rest with or without my consent.

I'm sorry to sound so negative; my life is not totally awful. The federal government provides safety nets for those of us who qualify for disability, so my life is pretty comfortable. I have a wonderful team of medical professionals and an even better support system—my friends, family, and church.

I took a series of biology courses in my late twenties for kicks and learned about genetic and inherited disorders. Information that I pulled from those classes led me to conclude that if my lupus were genetically inherited, I would have to have received it from two carriers (my parents) to get the full-blown disease. I don't know how scientifically sound that is, but hearing it gave me a sense of clarity. It took the blame from my hands. It made me feel like there was something greater and more vast at work. When I think of how vapid my concerns used to be in comparison, I'm led to believe there had to be some purpose in all of this.

The whole experience has given me greater empathy for others because I've been judged many times. People look at me, a person in her thirties, and wonder (out loud), "Why don't you just get better and get your life together?" I've learned patience for those who mean well by offering tons of advice about alternative treatments—every natural remedy, every new-age or biblical diet, and every exercise regimen under the sun. I am still learning acceptance. I've also learned to take each day one at a time while working on being in the here-and-now.

Fighting Lupus Battles

Commentary by Dr. Rosalind Ramsey-Goldman

If lupus is not treated during pregnancy, there is a significant risk that it will flare. In this case, it settled in the kidneys, causing permanent damage. Renal replacement (meaning either a dialysis machine or a new kidney, also known as a transplant) must be present to filter the body toxins that were previously filtered by the original kidney. The medications used when a kidney transplant is done usually also control lupus, making flares less likely. However, one needs to manage all of the pills and doctor visits on a set schedule to increase the chances that the transplanted kidney continues to work.

My Lupus Story

Gloria Morris

IN 2009, WHEN I was 28 years old and in my first semester of graduate school, I started experiencing leg spasms. I was treated by a chiropractor, but he didn't seem to heal or fix my issues at that time. My primary care physician completed several tests and found that I had rheumatoid arthritis. I was prescribed Celebrex. Later on that year, I was still having the leg spasms along with other issues such as fatigue, joint pain, stiffness, and inflammation around my heart. Then my primary care physician diagnosed me with systemic lupus erythematosus (SLE).

At that point I wasn't really having a lot of major issues, but in 2010 the lupus started affecting my heart more. I was experiencing sharp pains in my chest and occasional shortness of breath. The doctors determined the diagnosis as pericarditis. After I received treatment from cardiologists, my heart condition improved, and I went back to somewhat normal. However, my joint pain and frequent fatigue forced me to return to my rheumatologist. I was prescribed hydroxychloroquine (also known as Plaquenil), prednisone, and methotrexate. Those medications seemed to give me temporary relief.

In 2011 and 2012 I started having some major headaches, and I wasn't able to sit up for long periods of time. Then I started having seizures and memory loss. I experienced my first seizure after coming home from a doctor's appointment. I was hospitalized for two weeks, but they couldn't find anything that could have caused my seizures.

Fighting Lupus Battles

Six months later, I had another one. That time it was called a grand-mal seizure. I lost consciousness, and it was difficult for me to figure things out for myself. It was a very hard time for me. My doctors ran tests. It seemed that lupus had attacked my central nervous system and affected my brain, eyes, and hearing. I was having major headaches all the time. My headaches were so bad that I had to lie down. I was not able to sit up for much more than 15 minutes at a time. I couldn't sleep because my headaches were so severe. The lupus had attacked my eyes to the point where I was prohibited from driving. My ears were affected to the point where as of today I have a loss of hearing in both ears. My doctors were confused as to why I was having so many issues. So, I started participating in clinical trials, trying to find a way to control the lupus.

My rheumatologist recommended that I try Cytoxan infusions[1] for one year. It turned out that taking the infusions for only seven months alleviated some of the problems. I stopped having so much joint pain, and I experienced less swelling in my hands and feet. I had to have a spinal tap and take acetazolamide. The swelling in my brain went down, and the excessive fluid that was surrounding the brain decreased. But most importantly, those treatments slowed down the lupus, and I stopped having so many seizures.

Throughout my recovery, my lupus has been pretty stable. It has been so well controlled that I was able to earn my master's degree in business. I had a lot of support along the way. I am forever grateful for the support of my mother, medical team, and my lupus family here in Illinois.

---

1   Cytoxan, or cyclophosphamide, is used to treat certain cancers. It tends to work for many lupus patients as well. "When cyclophosphamide is used to treat cancer, it works by slowing or stopping the growth of cancer cells in your body. When cyclophosphamide is used to treat nephrotic syndrome (a disease that is caused by damage to the kidneys), it works by suppressing your body's immune system." (MedlinePlus)

My Lupus Story

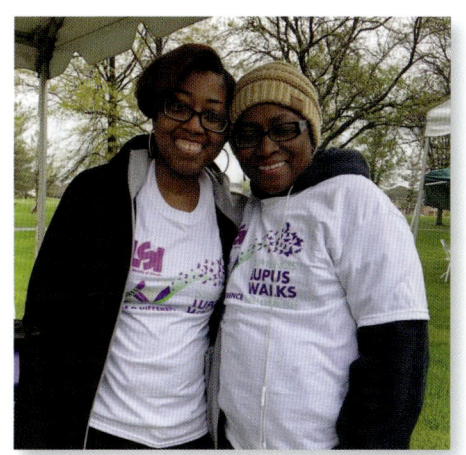

Gloria Morris with her mother, Roberta

Commentary by Dr. Rosalind Ramsey-Goldman

One of the most serious problems from lupus is when it affects the brain or nerves, causing a number of problems including severe headaches, seizures, difficulty thinking, and vision or hearing problems. Doctors have noted at least 19 different types of brain and nerve problems in patients with lupus. Sometimes, aggressive treatment is needed to get the symptoms under control and have them become less serious and hopefully go away completely.

Unwavering Faith and Courage

Sherry Y. Sims

I AM A SINGLE mother of three adult children—Letrianna, Robert, and Deloris Janette. I have found so much joy in raising them, and I cherish the comfort of having them closer to me now, more than ever.

Before being diagnosed with lupus, I had a lot of energy. I rode my bicycle, danced every chance I got, and traveled a lot. I was very outgoing—the life of the party. I loved gardening, socializing, volunteering, shopping, going to church, and I even held down five jobs at one time.

My life changed in 2009 when I was diagnosed with systemic lupus erythematosis . People told me that my condition was going to be hard and sometimes outright depressing. At first I didn't believe that would happen to me; I thought, *This too will pass.* As I slowly accepted my condition, I discovered they were right. I found out years later that lupus was not going anywhere. I have gone through some very dark times. I was even afraid I would give up, but with faith in God and the support of those who love me, I am STILL here.

Stress (good or bad) has been a factor in some of my flares. It seems that I can't win. I try to stay away from bad stresses. However, I must admit, I love the good ones, like playing with my grandkids or becoming overly excited when loved ones visit. I love having my kids around or people asking me to help them. Though my body reacts in a painful way once it is over, I always say it was worth it. It gives me a sense of feeling normal.

Unwavering Faith and Courage

Lupus can be very deceiving to the natural eye. People may actually look normal on the outside because lupus fights from within. It is a condition where the immune system not only fights off the bad germs, viruses, and bacteria, but it also attacks good parts of the body. There is no cure, just treatments and medications to help one manage. I remember someone made the statement to my son that I do not "look" sick. That made my son very angry. I told him to tell them I said thank you. I saw it as a compliment because the Lord knows I do not want to "look" sick.

Lupus can be a debilitating disease. Over the years I experienced extreme weakness, fatigue, arthritis in most joints, blood clots, muscle spasms, pneumonia, fibromyalgia, neuropathy, and now, medication-induced diabetes. The disease also affected my legs, hands, wrists, and shoulders. Arthritis in my knees and hips makes it hard to stand, walk, stoop, or bend. To control the pain and make daily living bearable, I take a total of ten pills per day and two injections weekly. As strange as it may seem, I prefer the injections because I do not have to eat or take meds continually throughout the day.

Lupus forces me to face several challenges. Because my condition requires that I have extensive periods of rest, it's difficult to manage a full-time job on a normal schedule. In order to make it through the week, I often have to alter my schedule by working two days and having two days off. I have fallen several times, so I cannot bathe unless someone else is with me. I have fallen asleep while cooking, so I feel it's too dangerous to try to prepare meals. I often need someone else to do that for me. Sometimes I am so weak I can't hold a fork to feed myself without dropping it. There are times I have to use a portable toilet due to not being strong enough to walk to the bathroom. I tire out instantaneously and can't move. My big toes both continue to feel frozen, and my feet sometimes feel like pins are going through them. Sometimes I am either too tired or weak to stay alert, and my attention span wanders. While talking, I might forget what I was talking about, or have trouble with what

Fighting Lupus Battles

words to use. Sometimes I have to end conversations prematurely because I get too exhausted to continue.

The best birthday present I have given myself was on November 21, 2015—going to my first support group meeting. I can truly say that bonding with people like me who understand, educate, and comfort one another has been instrumental in making sense out of this journey. We have celebrated our highs and our lows, and WE SHALL LIVE! These women have an unimaginable sense of inner strength and faith in God. I am so happy to be a part of such an edifying group of individuals.

I find joy in the comfort of my home by scrapbooking and doing various other crafts. To obtain a quality of life and be able to attend activities outside the home, I have been prescribed a power wheelchair. It has been instrumental in allowing me to return to work. The commute is a challenge, and the para-transit ride is extremely long. I am picked up two and a half hours before arrival time for work and sometimes spend up to four hours getting home.

I have been diagnosed as being totally disabled. Having my cousin, Shaun, as an advocate has surely made life easier. Having someone who loves and cares for me unconditionally has definitely helped me to know that I am not alone. I am moving through this nightmare with unwavering faith and courage because I have a place in this world, people to meet, knowledge to share, and family members who look up to me. My purpose is to be there, to conquer it all.

Unwavering Faith and Courage

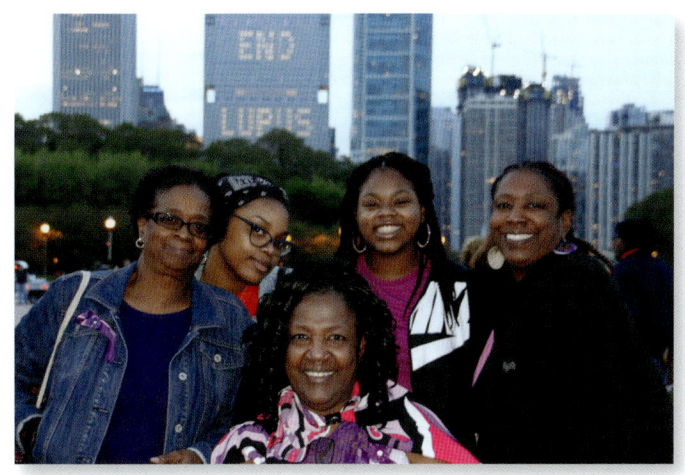

Sherry Sims, center

Commentary by Dr. Rosalind Ramsey-Goldman
Trying to find joy in the midst of adversity and celebrating what you *can* do rather than what you cannot do, fuels the courage and strength to be a lupus warrior.

Fighting Lupus Battles

Part I Summary

So what can I say?

Though many may live well with lupus, we know that it can be a mysterious, cruel, unpredictable, and potentially devastating disease. Since my near-death lupus flare, I have become very passionate about supporting the lupus community.

My passion has inspired us to do volunteer work with various lupus organizations. Cecil and I represent the Lupus Society of Illinois at various health fairs, participate in area lupus support groups, and speak at meetings of local organizations and churches.

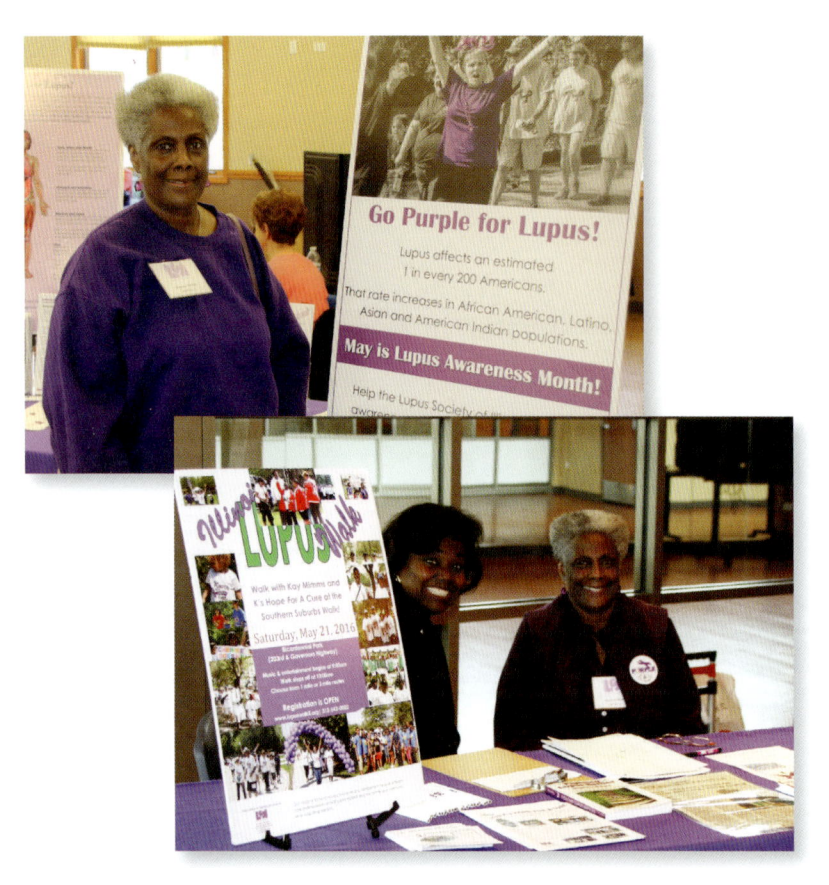

93

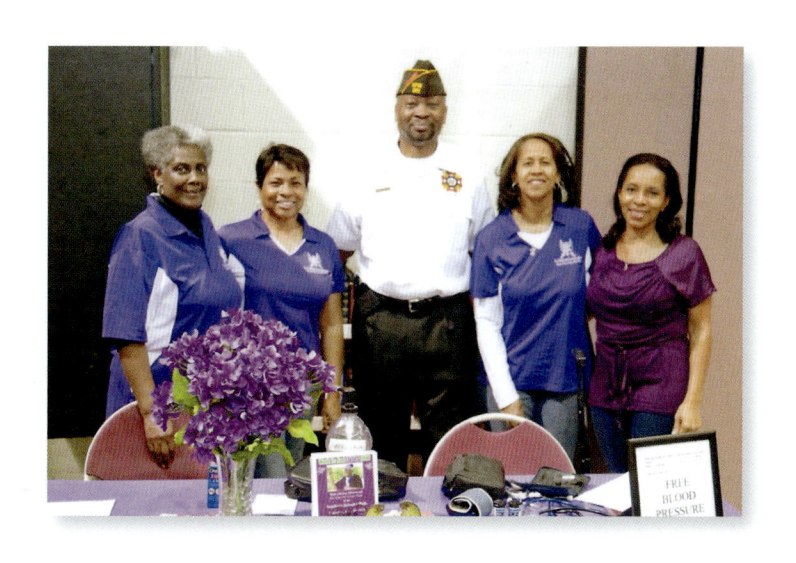

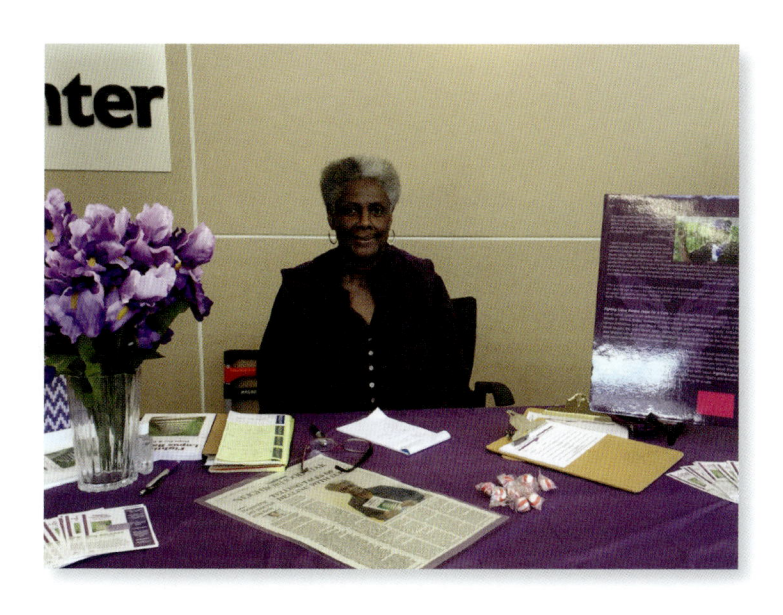

Fighting Lupus Battles

Serving as captains of Team K's Hope for a Cure in the Southern Suburbs Illinois Lupus Walk, sponsored by LSI, is another way that we help to support lupus warriors. Our ultimate goal is to help LSI and other organizations promote lupus awareness, support lupus patients, and raise funds for research that we hope will lead to more efficient diagnostic procedures, improved treatment plans, and a cure.

Cecil and Dana, our brother, captured images of participants in the Southern Suburbs Illinois Lupus Walk. Some family members in North Carolina supported the Charlotte Lupus Walk. The next few pages have collages with pictures of some of our strongest supporters.

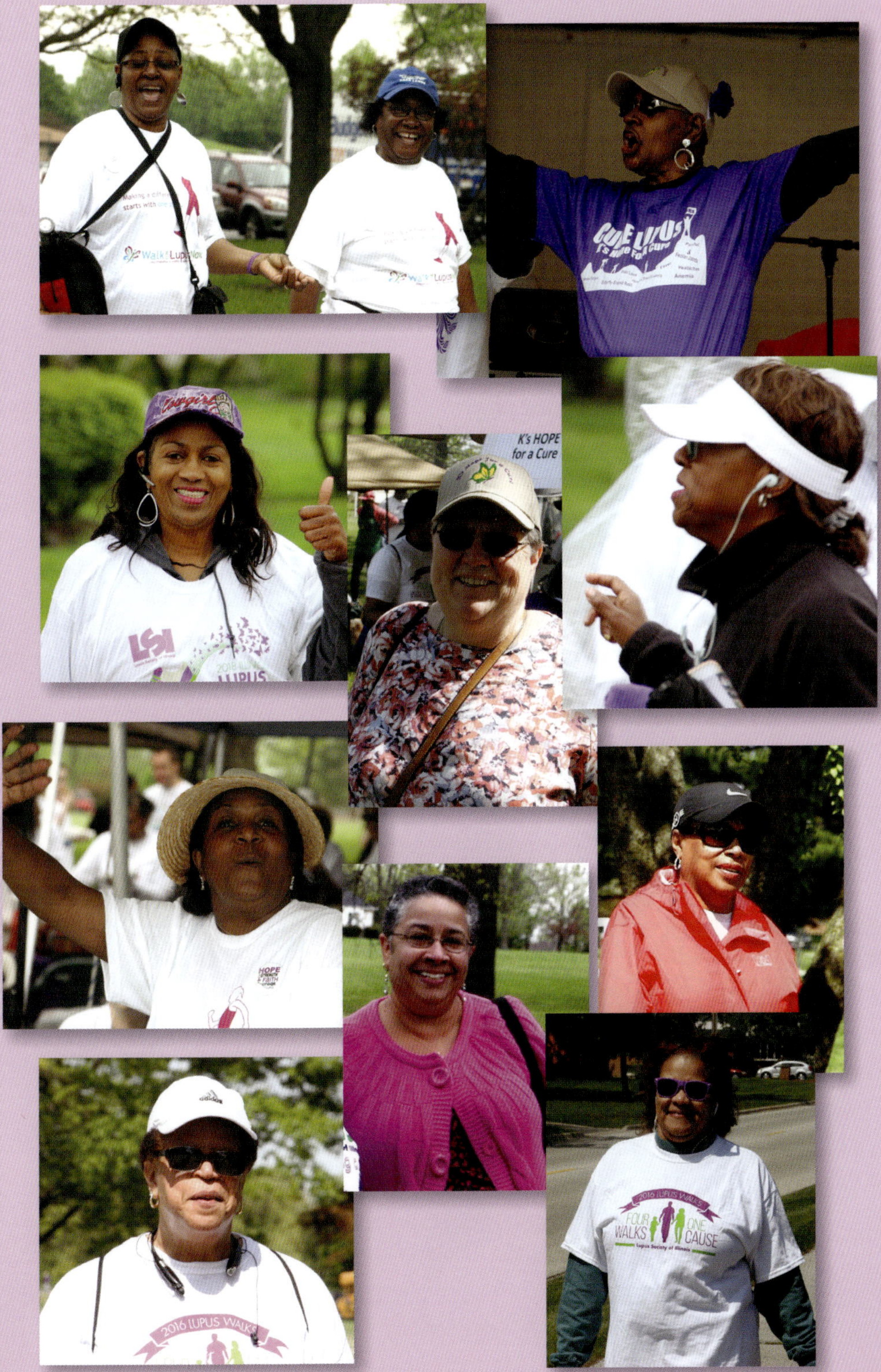
K's HOPE
for a Cure
2016 LUPUS WALKS
FOUR WALKS ONE CAUSE
2016 LUPUS WALKS

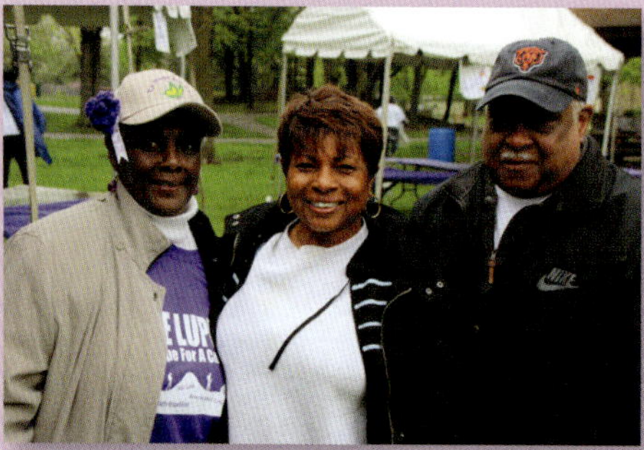

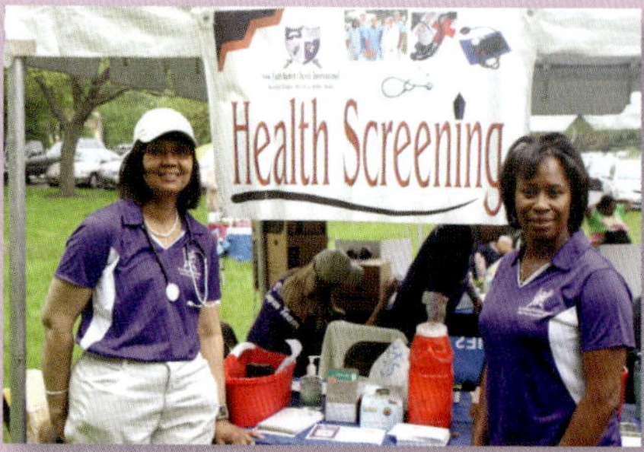
Health Screening

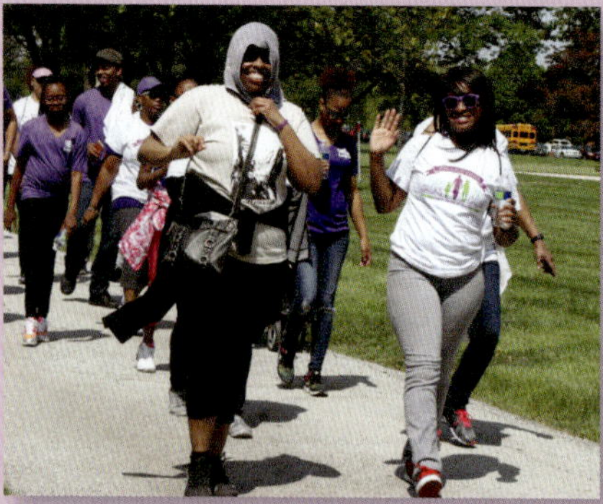

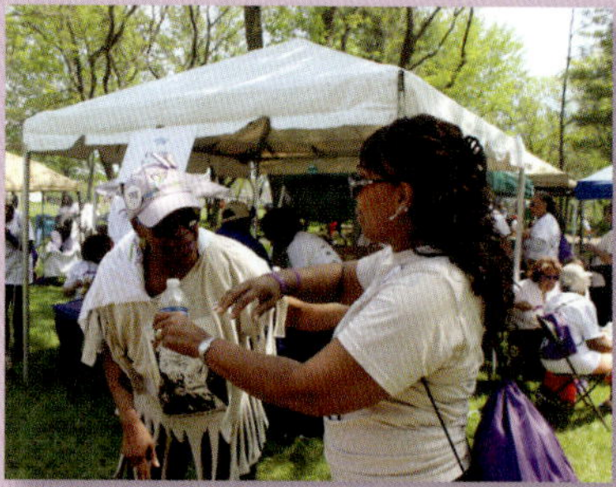

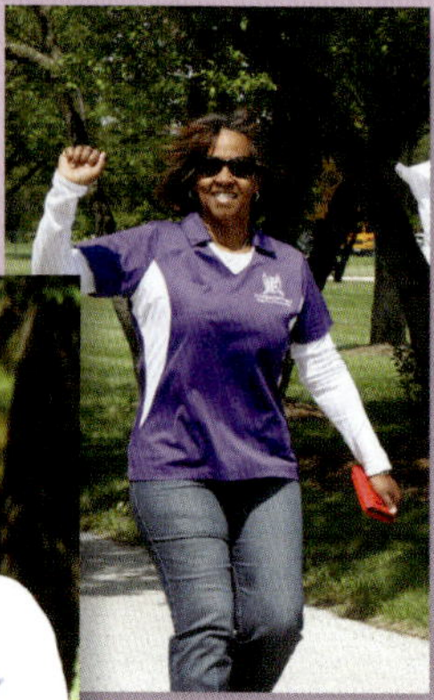

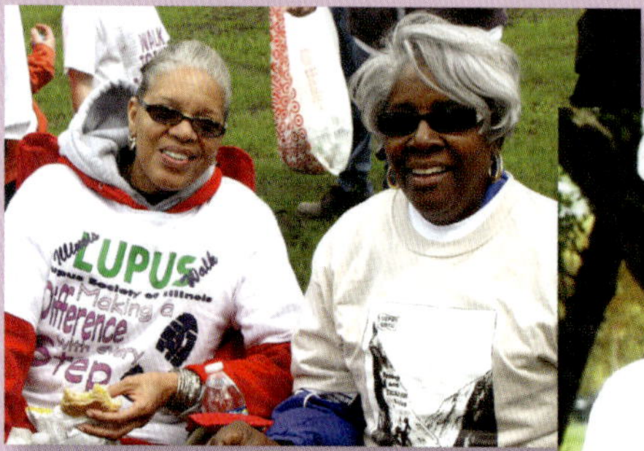
LUPUS
Lupus Society of Illinois
Making a
Difference

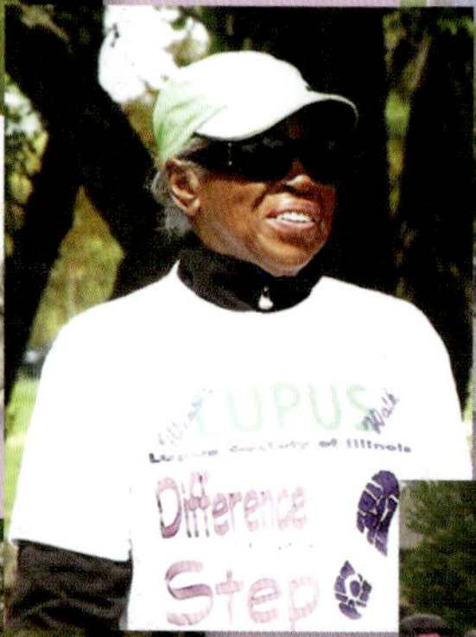
LUPUS
Difference
Step

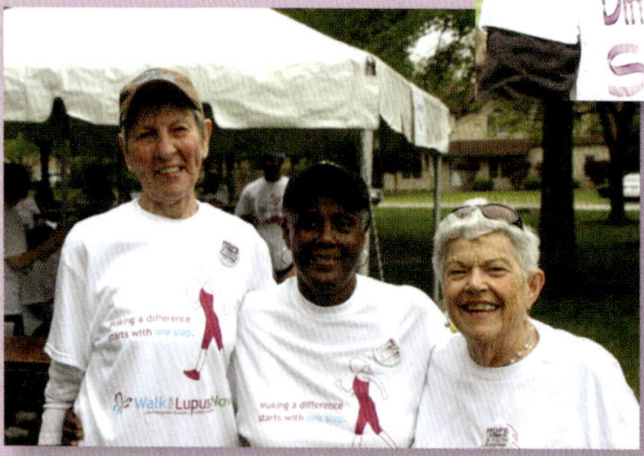

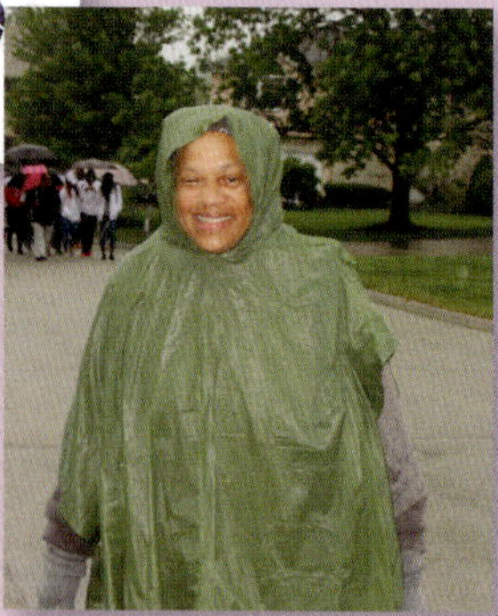

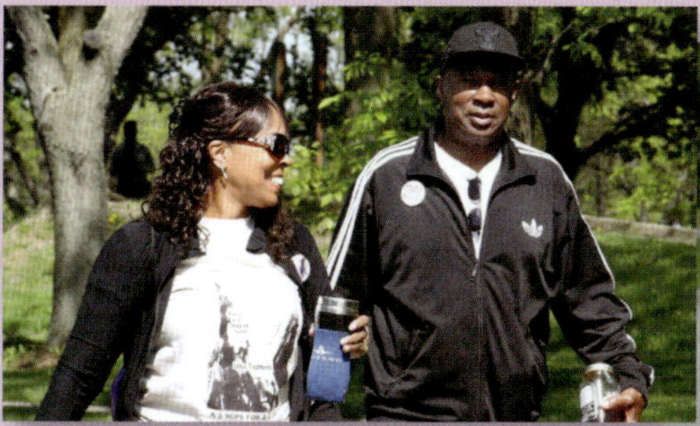

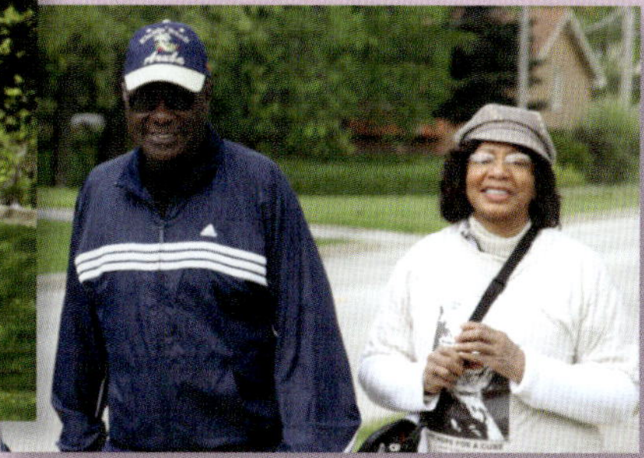

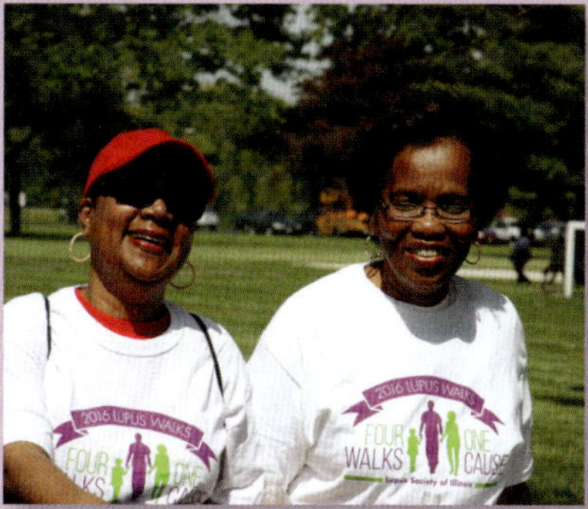
2016 LUPUS WALKS
FOUR
WALKS
ONE
CAUSE

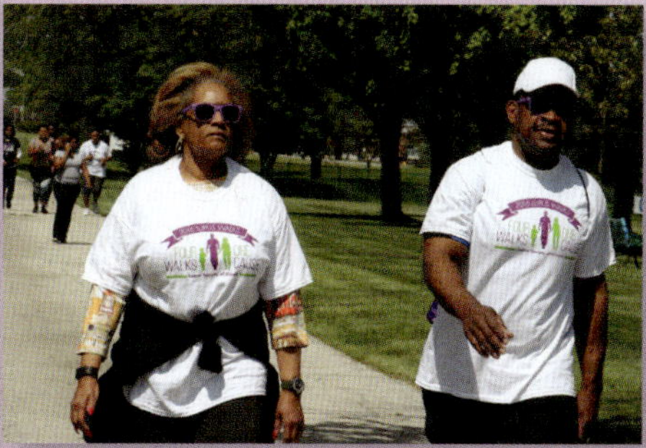

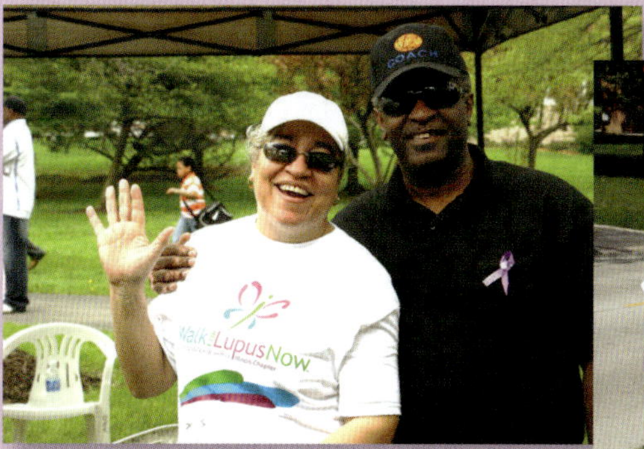
COACH
LupusNow

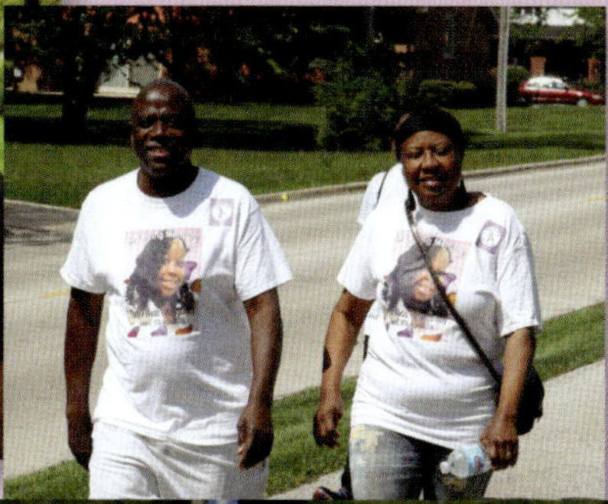

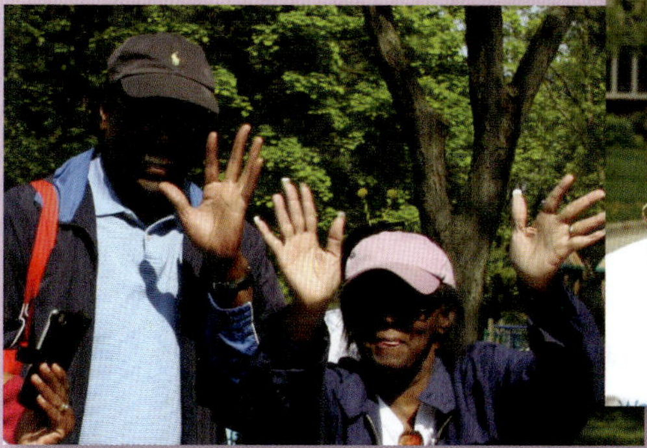

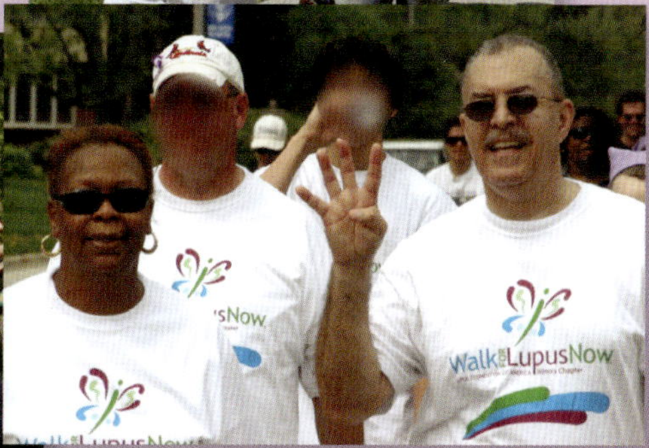
LupusNow

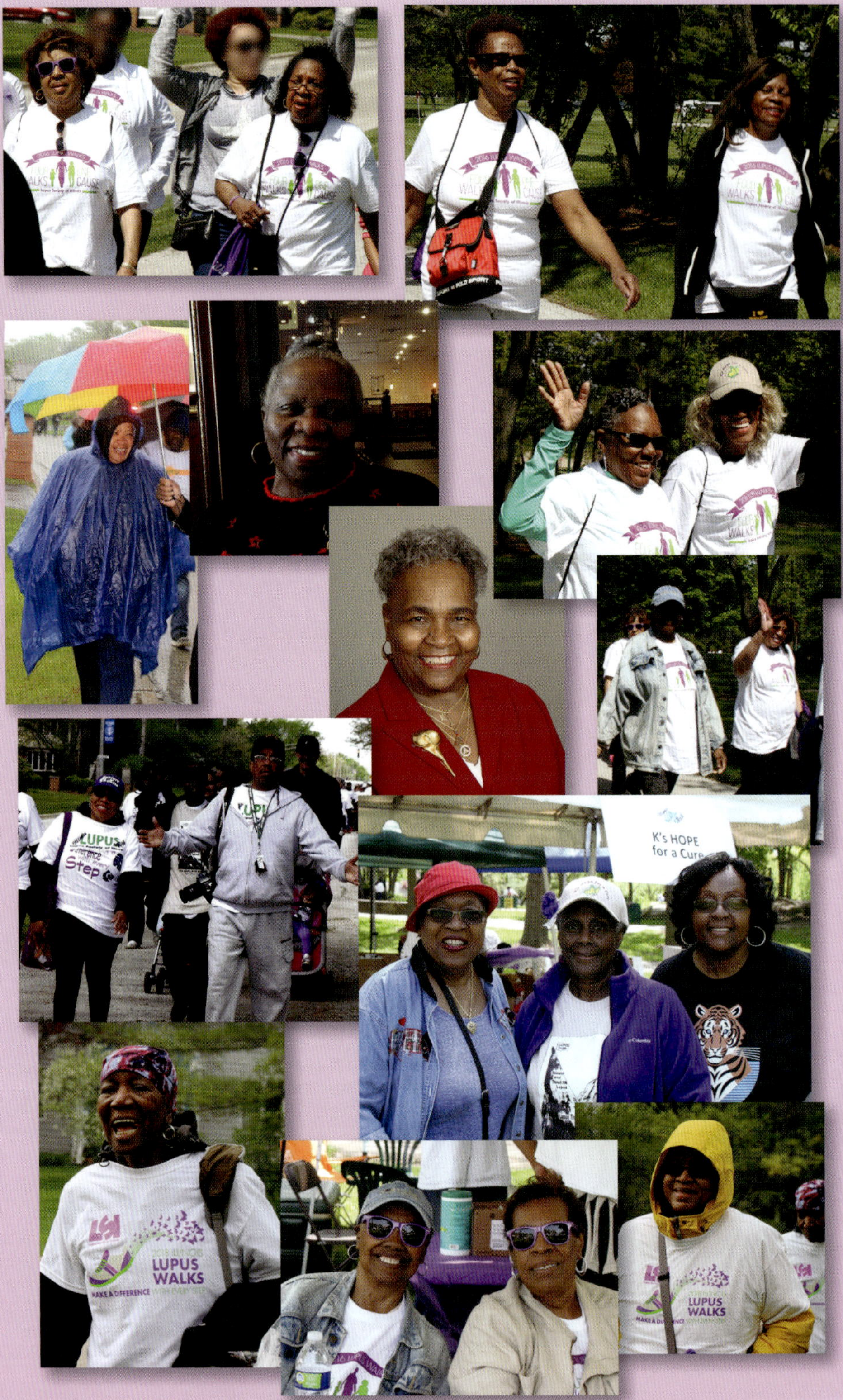
K's HOPE
for a Cure
LUPUS
WALKS
MAKE A DIFFERENCE
LUPUS
Step

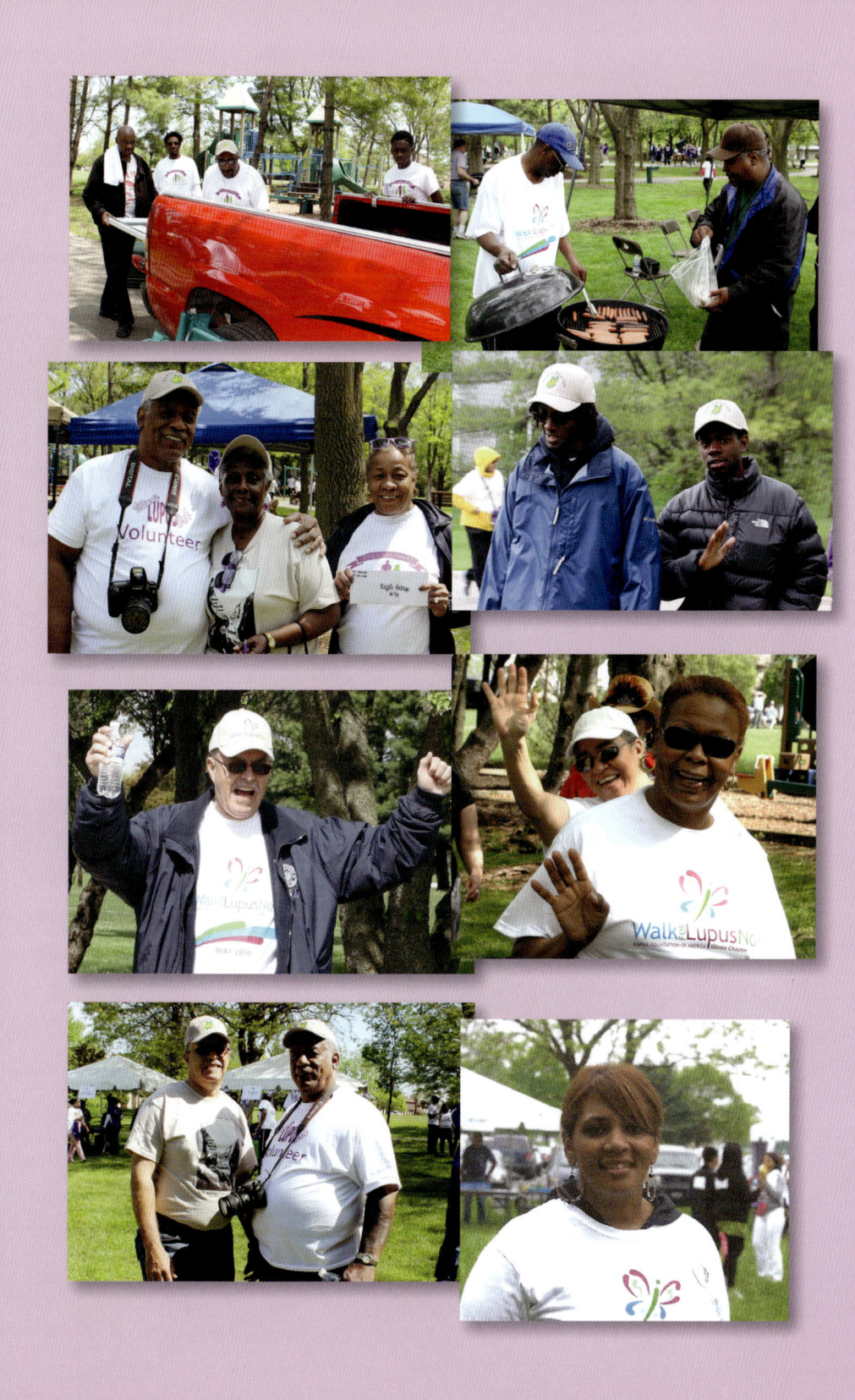

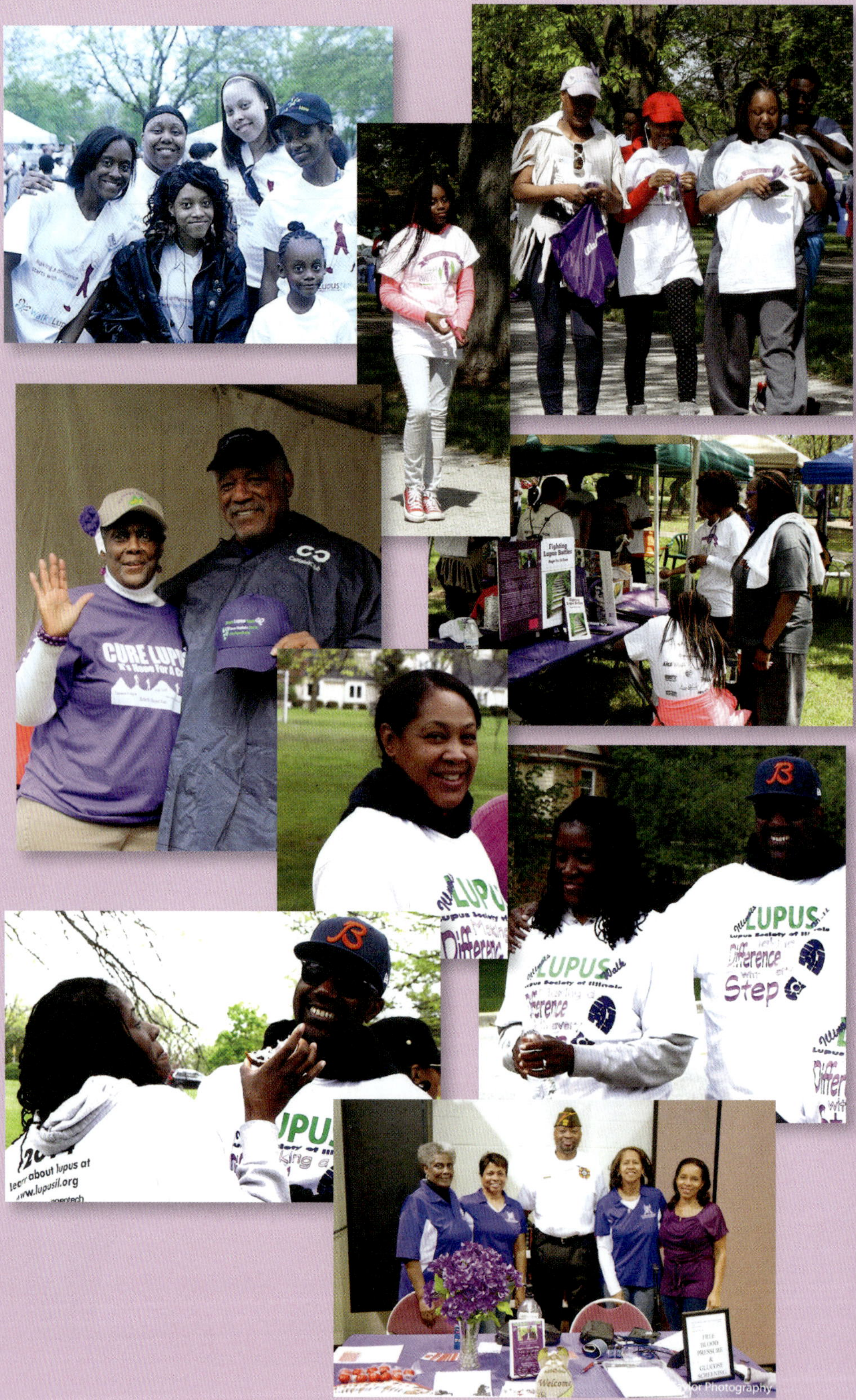
CORE LUPUS
LUPUS
Lupus Society of Illinois
Difference
Step
learn about lupus at
www.lupusil.org
Fighting Lupus Battles
FREE BLOOD PRESSURE & GLUCOSE SCREENING
Welcome

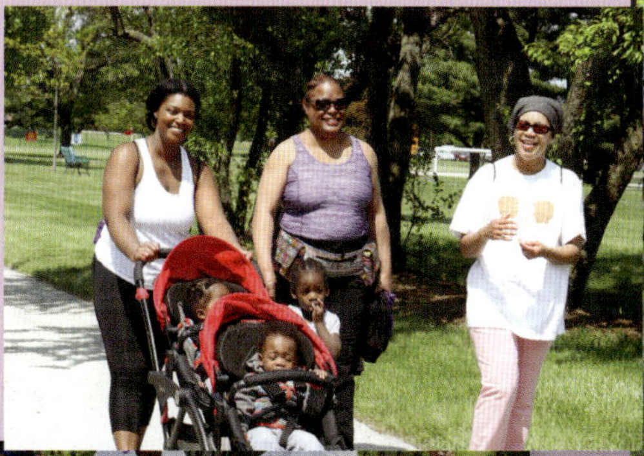

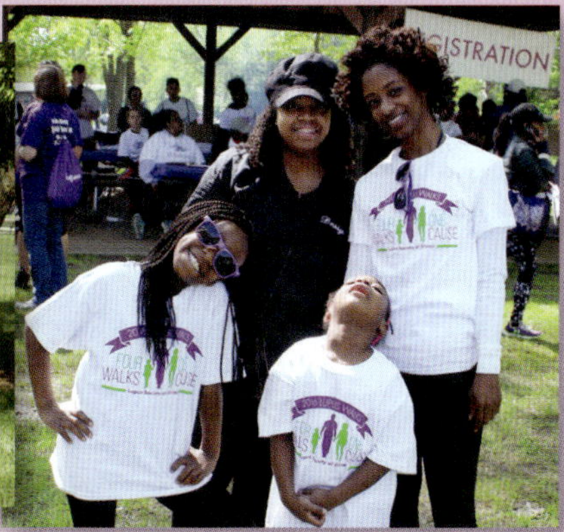
GISTRATION
WALKS
CAUSE

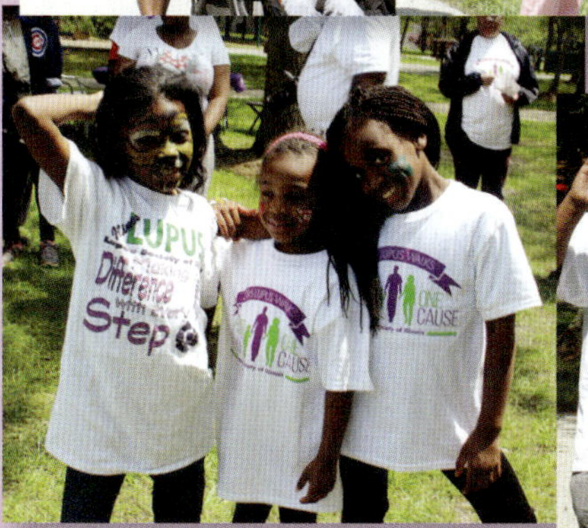
LUPUS
Difference
Step
ONE
CAUSE

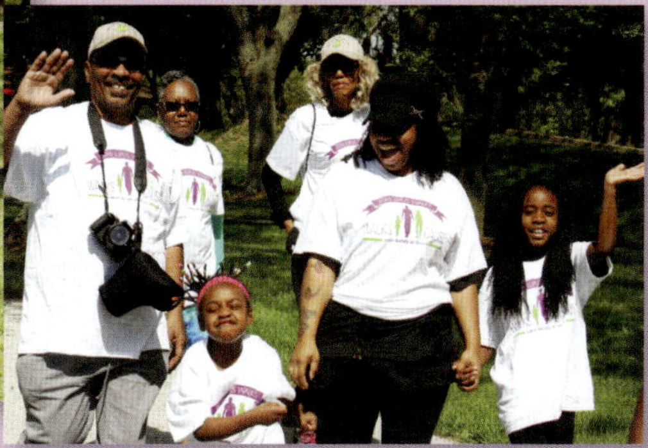

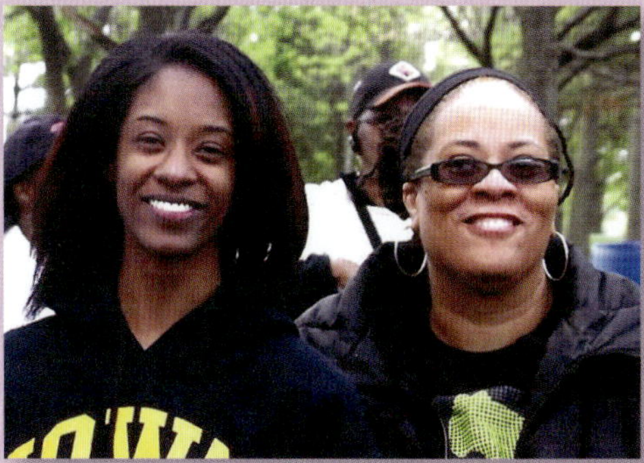

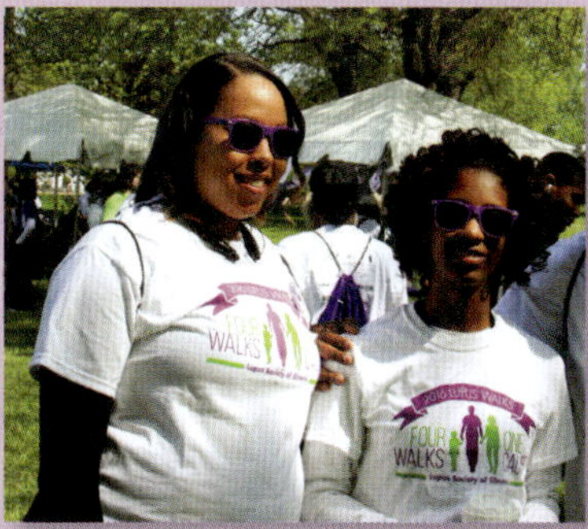
FOUR
WALKS

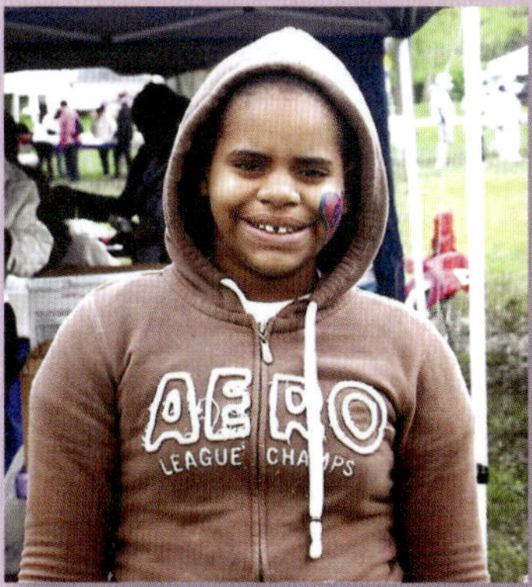
AERO
LEAGUE CHAMPS

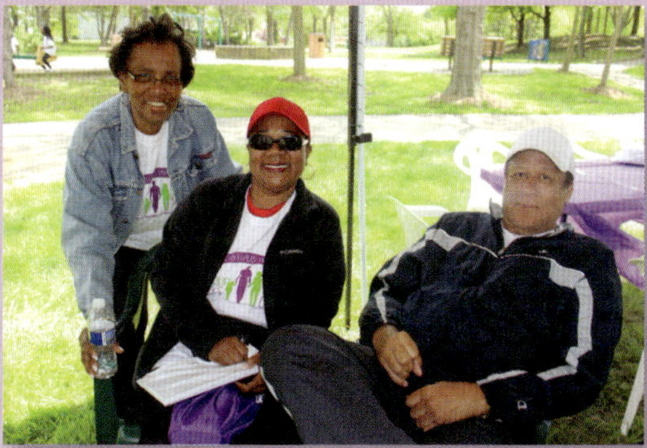

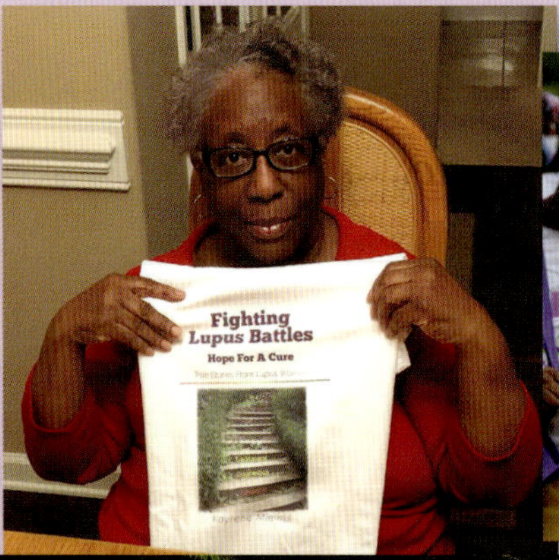
Fighting
Lupus Battles
Hope For A Cure

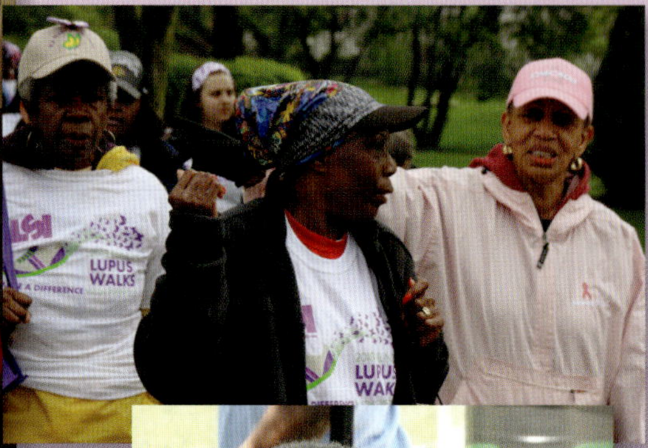
LUPUS
WALKS

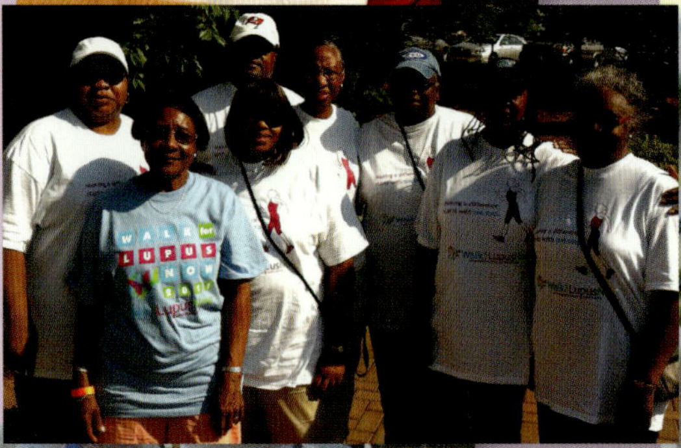

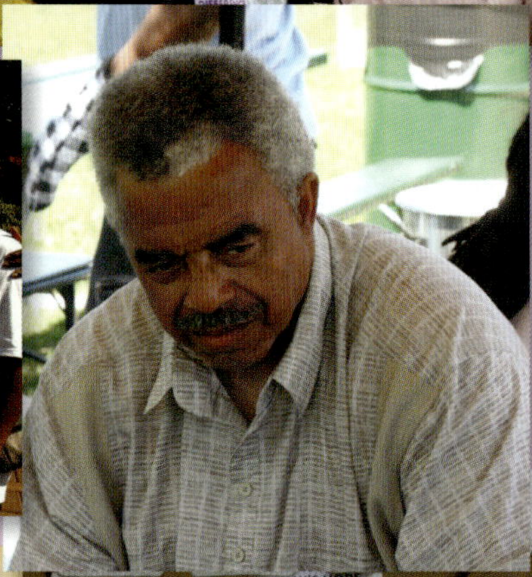

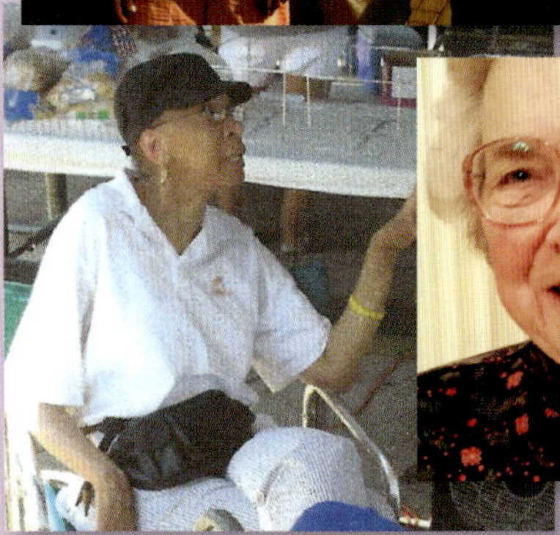

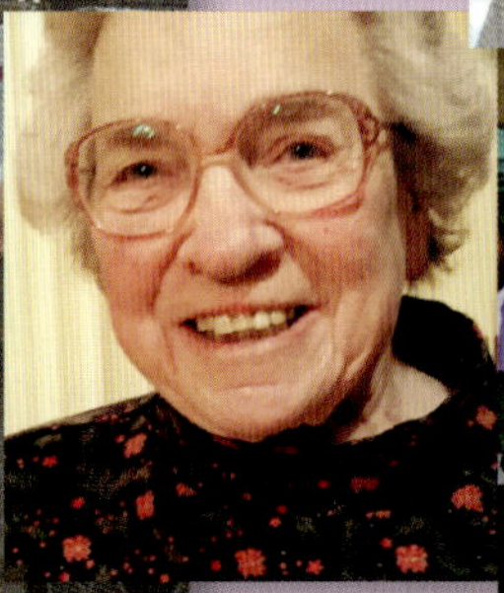

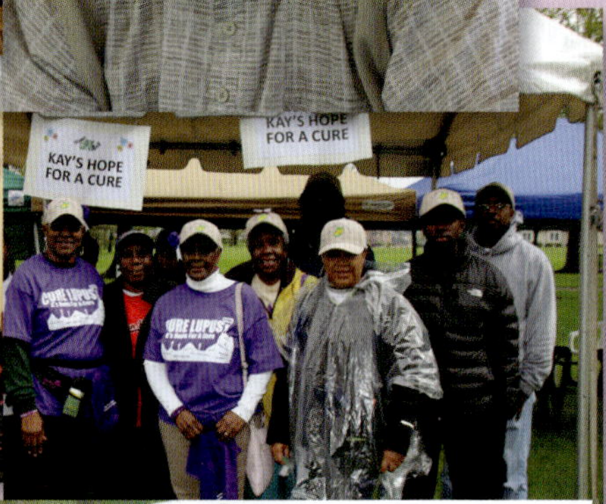
KAY'S HOPE
FOR A CURE
KAY'S HOPE
FOR A CURE

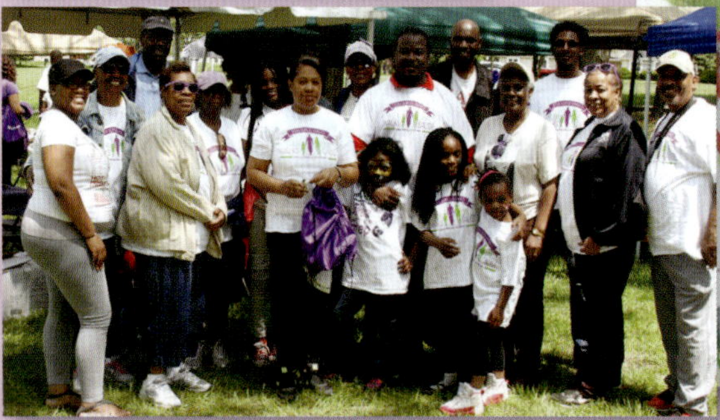

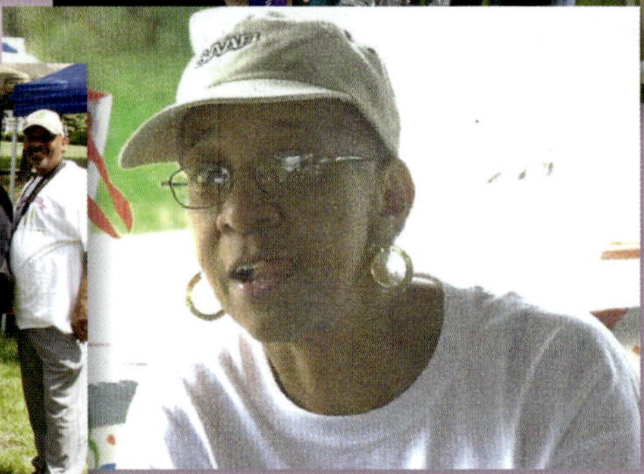

Part II

Finding Answers Through Research

THIS SECTION OF the book includes specific information about several clinical studies (clinical trials, or interventional; and observational, or non-interventional). "With research advances and a better understanding of lupus, the prognosis for people with lupus today is far brighter than it was in the past. It is possible to have lupus and remain active and involved with life, family and work. As current research efforts unfold, there is continued hope for new treatments, improvements in quality of life, and, ultimately, a way to prevent or cure the disease. The research efforts of today may yield the answers of tomorrow, as scientists continue to unravel the mysteries of lupus" (LSI website—About Lupus; Hope for the Future).

In this part, we'll learn about more lupus research projects from Kenneth and Ellyn Getz, Shanelle Gabriel, Dr. Rodlescia S. Sneed, Dr. Meenakshi Jolly, Dr. Kichul Ko, Dr. Rosalind Ramsey-Goldman, Dr. Teodora P. Staeva, Scott Hadly, and The Lupus Foundation of America. I'll also share my personal experiences in various clinical research studies.

What Clinical Research Means to You

Kenneth Getz, edited by Ellyn Getz

Kenneth Getz is an associate professor at Tufts University and the founder of CISCRP. Ellyn Getz is a senior manager in Development and Community Engagement for CISCRP.

THE CENTER FOR Information and Study on Clinical Research Participation (CISCRP) is a nonprofit organization dedicated to educating and informing the public, patients, medical/research communities, the media, and policymakers about clinical research and the role each party plays in the process. Our goal is to help you understand the clinical trial research process—including the risks and benefits of participating.

Have you ever taken an allergy medicine? Have you ever given your child a pain reliever? Perhaps you have a friend or a family member who is a lupus survivor. If so, you can thank a clinical research volunteer. Around the world people are living longer, healthier lives because someone they never met took part in a clinical research study. That's why at CISCRP we like to call research participants "medical heroes."

Most people don't understand what clinical research is all about. Some people are afraid to become participants because they may think clinical research volunteers are treated like "guinea pigs." They may be fearful because they've heard news stories about clinical trials that have gone wrong. They may still remember past abuses when protections were not in place. At CISCRP, we believe in "Education before Participation." We think that the more people understand research, the more empowered they'll feel to advocate for themselves and make informed decisions about their health.

What we learn from clinical research studies improves public health. It all starts with questions like these:

- Is there a better way to treat a disease like lupus?
- How well does a new drug work or not work?
- How do genes, hormones, and the environment affect lupus?
- What can be done to prevent and cure lupus?

Researchers can only answer these questions with the help of research volunteers.

What is Clinical Trial (Interventional) Research?

Clinical trial research is the scientific evaluation, based on the participation of study volunteers, to determine whether a medical treatment or approach is safe and effective. Clinical trials can be sponsored by the government, academic medical centers, pharmaceutical companies, biotechnology companies, or medical device companies.

Standard of Care

It's important to understand that being in a clinical trial is not the same as going to your doctor for care. When you go to your doctor, she'll give you a treatment that has already been tested and approved by the government. This is called "routine" or "standard of care." This is the care we know works for most people. An example of routine care is when a person breaks a bone and the doctor applies a cast. We know how it works for most people. An example of a clinical trial is checking whether a new drug works to prevent lupus flares.

The Importance of Diversity

You can't fully understand something by studying just one group of people. We know that things like gender, age, race, and ethnic background affect the way people respond to diseases and treatments. For example, women make up about nine out of every ten adults with lupus. "It's also more common in women of African-American, Hispanic, Asian, and Native-American descent than in Caucasian women" (Lupus Research Alliance). Children respond to drugs differently than adults. A lot of research involves healthy volunteers. Scientists need all different types of people to volunteer for research.

Clinical Trials: A Four-Phase Process

The whole clinical trial process has four phases. Completion of all four phases could take over ten years. During phase 1 studies, a drug is tested for the first time with a very small number of volunteers. Often, the participants are healthy volunteers. The goal of these trials is to learn about safe dosage. How does it work in the body? Is it harmful?

In phase 2 studies, researchers begin to understand how well a drug works and if it is safe. Like phase 1, safety is still the main goal. Phase 2 studies look to answer basic questions such as: how much should people take? What are the usual side effects? Only about one-third of drugs that enter clinical testing ever successfully complete phase 2 and progress to larger, phase 3 studies.

Phase 3 provides hard facts about a drug from a large group of patients. At this stage, researchers may check the drug's safety and how well it works in different groups of patients. Another goal of the trial may be to compare the new drug with an already approved drug.

Phase 4 studies happen after a treatment has been approved by the Food and Drug Administration (FDA). They usually involve large numbers of patients who are regularly taking a medicine. Phase 4 studies look at real-world experience and check to see if the drug works well over a long period of time.

Members of the Study Team

Research involves many people who do different things. Like members of a sports team, clinical trials have coaches, players, and officials, and each person has an important role to play.

The Principal Investigator (PI) is like the team manager who directs the team. The PI is responsible for organizing and leading the study as well as recording and studying the data. Like a team manager, the PI follows a playbook, which is called the study protocol. The protocol is a set of instructions that everyone in the game must follow. It's the plan for how the study will be carried out.

The research staff members are like assistant managers who help the PI. The clinical research coordinator (CRC) handles the day-to-day activity at the research site. He or she has easy access to the PI and is the main contact for volunteers. If you have questions about the trial or your health, ask the CRC.

Referees help protect the safety of volunteers by making sure teams follow the rules. The referees review the study before it starts, give you all the information, and keep you safe. The numbers and types of referees involved in a trial depend on the research that is being conducted. Referees from the federal government are also involved. Regulatory bodies review studies, inspect research centers, and monitor research groups. The regulatory bodies have the final say in whether or not a treatment is approved.

Every clinical trial is reviewed, approved and watched over by an independent local committee called an institutional review board, or IRB. It's the law. IRBs consist of at least five members who come from various backgrounds and have professional experience relevant to the study. At least one member should be a scientist, and at least one must focus on nonscientific concerns. In addition, one member of the IRB must be a community member who is not affiliated with the organization that is conducting the study. Ideally,

What Clinical Research Means to You

the members of the board should be diverse in gender, race, and culture. The IRB makes sure a trial is ethical and fair and that there is not too much risk to the volunteers. During the trial, researchers must let the IRB know if there are any changes in the study plan or if volunteers experience serious injuries or side effects. The IRB can end a trial if it feels volunteers are not safe.

The most important members of the team are the research volunteers. Volunteers are like the players on the field. Without them, research can't happen. We need all different types of people to participate in clinical research.

Eligibility Criteria

Just like in sports, clinical trials have *eligibility criteria*. In sports, the coaching staff members draft players who can play certain positions. In clinical trials, the research team has a list of requirements for the participants. The guidelines help determine who can or can't be in a study. Eligibility criteria protect people if a trial might be too risky for them. This helps researchers get results that are accurate and meaningful.

Let's assume the coaches say you're eligible to play. Now you need to ask several questions. First, do I choose to play? Well, that depends, right? You can't say whether or not you want to participate without understanding the rules of the game. What are your responsibilities as a player? How long will the game last? What are the risks and benefits of playing? What are you going to get in exchange for playing? Everyone has the chance to participate in research; you just have to find the study that is right for you.

Informed Consent

The *informed consent* process is designed to answer all these questions and is required by the FDA and IRB. This is one of the most important parts of research, and it's a term you're going to hear a lot. Before any volunteer can participate in a trial, he or she must read, understand, and sign the informed consent form.

Fighting Lupus Battles

This is a long form that lists your rights as a volunteer. It includes detailed facts about the trial. It describes your job as a volunteer and any procedures or tests you'll need to have. It will warn you about any known or unknown side effects of the study drug. It describes the benefits of participating in the trial. By signing the form you're saying that you understand the trial and are agreeing to do what the study asks.

The informed consent form is a complex document. The study staff should go through it carefully with you and answer all your questions. You should never feel rushed or pressured to sign the form. It is important to note that the IRB can ask the researcher to translate the informed consent form to a language the volunteer speaks.

A Study Volunteer's Bill of Rights

As a research volunteer, you have rights. You have the right to understand the purpose, benefits, risks, and side effects of the clinical trial. You have the right to ask any questions and discuss any concerns with the research staff at any time during the trial. You also have the right to full, complete, and clear answers. Most importantly, you have the right to quit the trial at any time for any reason. You are a volunteer and are free to leave the trial if you choose to. The research staff will help you do this safely!

Understanding the Study Design

Scientists set up their studies so that their research will be fair. They also want their research to be accurate and unbiased. In other words, they don't want their own ideas about what they think should happen in a trial to influence the results.

To set up fair and unbiased studies, volunteers may be split into different study groups. This is usually done by chance using a computer program and is similar to a coin toss. The researcher and the volunteer DO NOT get to decide which group the volunteer will be in. This is called a *randomized* study. Sometimes researchers will go a step further and *blind* a study. This means

What Clinical Research Means to You

that neither the volunteer nor the researcher know which treatment the volunteer is receiving.

In some trials, researchers will use a *placebo*. A placebo looks like medicine but has no medicine in it. Sometimes the placebo is referred to as a "sugar pill." What's interesting is that even though the placebo has no medicine in it, there are times when people who are taking a placebo improve or feel better during a trial. This is called the *placebo effect*. As a clinical research volunteer, even if you are on a placebo, you will be closely monitored.

Possible Benefits and Risks

Deciding whether or not to participate in a clinical research trial is an important, personal decision. It is good to talk to your friends and family about the study. They can help you come up with questions to ask your doctor about the study. They can also support you while you participate. In the end, it is your job to make the final decision. Some of the reasons why people say they get involved in research trials include:

- to gain access to brand new therapies that are not yet available on the market
- to advance science and help others with their condition
- because the research staff will observe your health closely

- because some trials pay for volunteers' time, commitment, and travel costs. Not all trials pay, and if they do the amounts vary widely. Getting paid should never be your only reason for volunteering.

The clinical trial research process is highly regulated. Experienced professionals manage it, and it has many built-in safeguards to help ensure a safe and positive volunteer experience. Although there is promise and hope for volunteers, even the best-run clinical trials are never completely free of risk. Possible risks include:

- Physical—You may not get better. There might be some undesirable side effects that may make you feel uncomfortable.
- Emotional—Some clinical trials may ask you to take a quality-of-life survey to see how you are doing, and some of the questions can be upsetting or cause distress.
- Financial—there could be out of pocket expenses such as parking, childcare, and unpaid time off of work.
- Privacy and confidentiality—usually your health information is private. When you agree to participate in research, you are giving permission for researchers to collect information about you. Researchers must follow rules that protect your privacy and your information. It's important that all of your doctors know if you are in a clinical trial.

Education Before Participation

If you decide to join a study, you should feel confident that you have made an informed choice. You should feel comfortable that the trial staff will support you and answer all your questions.

- Do your homework. Learn about the trial and ask questions. Read all the information provided by the study staff. You may even go online to research the treatment being studied.

What Clinical Research Means to You

- Take your time. There is absolutely nothing wrong with asking a researcher to slow down or explain something using simpler words.

- Ask questions. Talk about your concerns with the study staff, your doctor, your friends, and family. Bring a friend or family member to study visits so they can ask questions too. Tape record your visits or take notes so you can refer to the information later and follow up with questions as needed.

If you're interested in learning more about participation opportunities, you can get information from your doctor, a local research center, disease advocacy groups, medical journals, and conferences. There are also websites devoted to clinical trials like www.clinicaltrials.gov, www.ciscrp.org, and www.centerwatch.com. Feel free to give us a call at 617-725-2750. CISCRP provides a free search service designed to help people find trials that might be right for them. You may also talk to your doctor, research site, friends and family to help find resources for you.

Research volunteers truly are "medical heroes." Without them, medical science cannot move forward. Thank you for taking time to learn about the clinical research process. Finally, thanks to the millions of people who give the gift of participation in clinical trials each year.

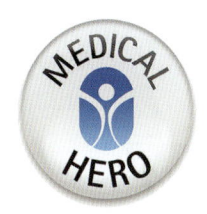

Interview with Shanelle Gabriel

Ellyn Getz

Title of the study or trial; purpose/objective of the research:

I participated in an investigational study that tested a version of a new lupus drug.

How were you introduced to the study? What motivated you to participate?

Originally I didn't want to go on the new drug. I had been seeing the same rheumatologist since 2004 when I was diagnosed with a mild-to-moderate case of lupus. I tried "light" medications when not much was happening and stronger ones when everything was failing. But there was nothing in between. I tried so many different drugs. I had even been on steroids for a long time; that wasn't ideal for me. My rheumatologist introduced me to the study.

My rheumatologist was very open while explaining the whole study process. She walked me through what would happen if things didn't go well, if my body didn't love it, and how I might react to it. She talked to me about what might happen and made me feel more comfortable about participating in a trial that was experimental.

I still had reservations. I've never had kids, and I didn't want to do anything that would affect my ability to get pregnant. On the other hand, I thought, how could I expect new drugs to help if I don't try

Interview with Shanelle Gabriel

something? So I did some digging and searching and saw that I could try something. I felt more comfortable after I did my own research into the potential risks and the benefits.

I thought the new lupus drug might be a good middle point to manage the flares. I thought it was a good option to see if the new drug worked. So I got involved out of frustration, not desperation, and with the possibility that something good could come out of it. That possibility motivated me to go ahead and try it.

What did the trial entail?

My rheumatologist is a part of a teaching hospital in New York, and I was used to traveling there. I just needed to travel there a bit more often to meet the study requirements and do blood work.

I had to learn how to take the medication myself. It required injection. I had to inject myself. The medication had to be taken and recorded at a certain time. I had to answer questions every week. It was mainly understanding what I was doing and the reasons behind it.

The study's team members were very thorough, but they explained things on a general level. I consider myself a more advanced patient, and I ask a lot of questions so as not to omit anything. I didn't know who else was in the study. I don't know if anyone else came in for study visits at the same time I did. I had to work around my work schedule—luckily, the study team was very accommodating.

Summary

I was involved in the study for a few months, and I felt comfortable participating. The drug was ultimately approved. I am on the medication now, and it is helping. It's still new, so I'm still keeping track of what I look and feel like. I continue to see my rheumatologist for regular check-ups. Something else that is helpful to me is fitness. I swear by it and wonder if there's a connection to the severity of the lupus symptoms. I know other lupus warriors can feel achy, and

Fighting Lupus Battles

there can be a lot of pain. I wonder if the severity can be a result of inactivity before the diagnosis. I'm blessed to know how to dial back. I've never stopped exercising and being active. There are some serious or severe things that have happened, but exercise helps me function. I don't run as much; I lift weights, do some high-intensity interval training (HIIT-style), pole dance, and spin.

Anyone who is trying to figure out if a clinical trial is right for you should ask the right questions. If you don't know something, ask. Don't just think that there's a reason why you shouldn't know. Let them answer your questions.

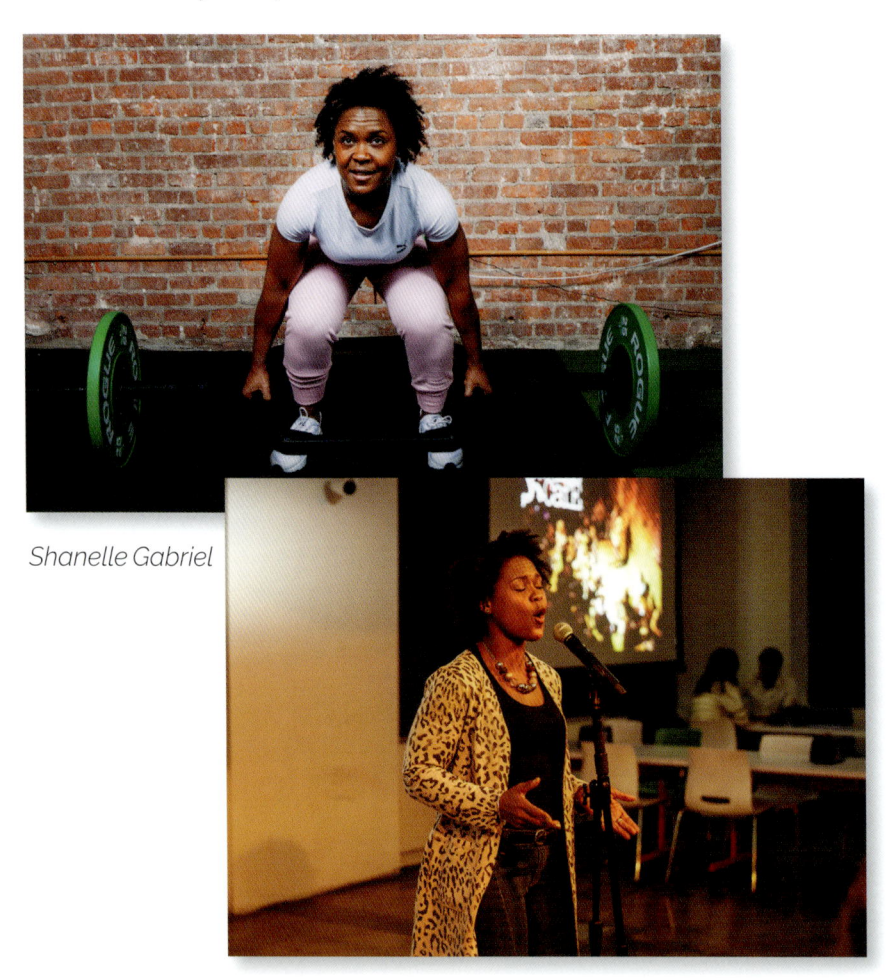

Shanelle Gabriel

African-American Participation in Lupus Clinical Research: Why it Matters

Rodlescia S. Sneed, PhD, MPH

Dr. Sneed is an assistant professor in the Department of Family Medicine, Division of Public Health, College of Human Medicine at Michigan State University.

SYSTEMIC LUPUS ERYTHEMATOSUS is a chronic autoimmune disease that can affect numerous systems of the body, including the kidneys, joints, brain, and blood vessels. Although anyone can get the disease, it most often affects women. Women from ethnic minority groups are more commonly impacted by lupus than Caucasian women. African-American women are three times more likely to develop lupus than Caucasian women. Further, when African-American women are diagnosed with lupus, it occurs at much younger ages, and it is much more severe than it is in Caucasian women. Researchers do not fully understand why lupus is more common and severe for African Americans; however, many believe that a combination of genetic, hormonal, and environmental factors may play a role.

There are very few drugs available to treat lupus. Most treatments focus on preventing/treating disease flares, minimizing pain, and reducing swelling. The best hope for better lupus treatment involves the development and testing of new drugs that, if effective, can be combined with existing treatments to provide the most effective and comprehensive therapy possible. There are several new drugs on the horizon that could be of benefit to individuals living with lupus. New drugs, however, cannot be developed and

Fighting Lupus Battles

utilized without research volunteers—individuals who have lupus and agree to be involved in lupus clinical trials.

Clinical trials are important for discovering new treatments. They help researchers to figure out which drugs work, the types of side effects that these drugs may have, and if the benefits of a new drug outweigh its potential risks. Countless people have benefited from treatments that were developed because other people were willing to participate in clinical trials that were used to identify and test newer, more effective therapies.

Clinical trials have several phases. In phase I, researchers evaluate the safety of a drug in a small group of people. They conduct research to determine the safest dose of a drug and to identify its potential side effects. In phase II, a drug is given to a larger group of people. In this phase, researchers still test for safety and also begin to evaluate the drug's effectiveness. In phase III, a drug is given to an even larger number of people (think thousands) to even further evaluate its effectiveness. In this phase, the drug is compared to other commonly used treatments, and researchers continue to collect information on how to most safely use the drug.

Although African-American communities are most impacted by lupus, African Americans are much less likely to participate in clinical trials than Caucasians. This difference is likely due to historical mistrust surrounding research in African-American communities. The legacy of the Tuskegee Syphilis Study, an unethical research experiment conducted solely among African-American men in the rural south from 1932 to 1972, has greatly impacted how research is viewed in African-American communities.

Without African-American participation in clinical trials, it will be difficult to reduce the large racial disparities in lupus-related outcomes. If African Americans do not participate in trials, it means that they are not likely to receive any of the benefits from lupus

African-American Participation in Lupus Clinical Research

research advances. One of the major goals of any research study is to take the findings from that study and then attempt to generalize those findings to the larger population. It is important for African Americans to be represented in clinical trials to be sure that any findings that come from trials can actually be applied to African Americans. Drugs that have been only tested among Caucasians may not be as effective or have the same side effects among African Americans. If African Americans fail to participate in trials, it is very difficult to know if drugs will work in the same way as they do for Caucasians and other groups. A lack of clinical trial data for African Americans means that physicians have less information to guide them in treating African American patients. A drug is less valuable if the studies that led to its development do not include the full range of individuals who might one day receive that drug when it becomes widely available.

For people with lupus, participating in a clinical trial may have direct benefits. Clinical trials can help people with lupus to feel empowered. When you participate in a clinical trial, you are becoming an active participant in your own healthcare decisions. Participating in a trial also gives people with lupus access to the newest medications that may be available. For someone with a particularly complex disease experience, such new medications may provide greater benefit than existing drugs. Involvement with a clinical trial also provides access to some of the best doctors and medical care available. The researchers who conduct clinical trials are widely known for their disease-related expertise. People who participate in clinical trials are closely monitored and receive cutting-edge medical care. This is care that, for many people, might not be available otherwise.

Participating in a clinical trial may also help the families of people living with lupus. Many researchers believe that genes play a role in the development of lupus, as lupus tends to run in families. A person is much more likely to develop lupus if there is a family

Fighting Lupus Battles

member who also has the disease. This is especially true for children and siblings. Thus, a person with lupus who participates in a clinical trial may help to develop a drug or treatment that benefits a close relative.

Finally, clinical trials help to move science forward. This means that even if direct benefits do not emerge for the individual, clinical trials have a larger benefit to society. Each person who participates in a clinical trial today helps to make things better for future lupus warriors who will battle this disease.

By participating in clinical trials, African-American patients with lupus can help themselves, their families, and society at large. Advances in science and treatment do not happen without research. Given the large differences in lupus-related outcomes for African Americans compared to other racial/ethnic groups, clinical trials are important. Without them, we can never hope to reduce the racial differences in treatment outcomes for African Americans.

My Lupus Research Experiences

Kayrene Mimms

BEFORE I WAS diagnosed with lupus, I never considered being a research participant. My reservations revolved mainly around safety, privacy, confidentiality, research objectives, and reliability of results. My attitude changed after being diagnosed with lupus and going through a near-death experience. I had suffered with lupus-like symptoms at different times throughout my life. I was even evaluated for lupus twice, and it was determined that I did not have it. I was almost sixty years old before I received an accurate diagnosis—systemic lupus erythematosus.

I was disappointed and confused. All kinds of thoughts ran through my mind. *What caused me to have lupus? What made the doctors think I had lupus in the first place? Why did it take so long to get an accurate diagnosis? Why did the lupus attack my skin and eyes first? Why did it attack my lungs and heart? Two of my nieces, Barbara and Noel, died from lupus. Could it be hereditary?* Thank God that by the time I was diagnosed, clinical research (clinical trials and observational studies) had produced a wealth of knowledge about successful lupus treatment plans that included prednisone and Cytoxan. These treatments saved my life. Being able to overcome the near-death flare convinced me that lupus research is critical for answering the questions I had. I felt it was my duty to get involved in clinical lupus studies on some level.

Clinical studies involve research using human volunteers, called participants, to add to medical knowledge. The two main categories of clinical research are clinical trials (interventional) and observational studies (non-interventional).[1] In a clinical trial, "participants receive specific interventions according to the research plan or protocol created by the investigators. These interventions may be medical products, such as drugs or devices; procedures; or changes to participants' behavior, such as diet."[2] In an observational study, "individuals are observed or certain outcomes are measured. No attempt is made to affect the outcome (for example, no treatment is given)."[3]

As I learned about lupus—the difficulty of obtaining an accurate diagnosis, not knowing the cause, its potentially devastating effects on the body, the side effects of some treatments, and the fact that there is no cure—I gained a greater respect for lupus research and its participants. I believe that research is a major avenue that will lead to prevention, earlier diagnosis, better treatment plans, and eventually, a cure. When the opportunity to participate in several observational studies arrived, I jumped on board.

The studies in which I have participated include Fatigue and Lifestyle Physical Activities and SLE Study; SOLVABLE Heart and Bone Study; Systemic Lupus Erythematosus International Collaborating Clinics (SLICC)'s Registry for Atherosclerosis in SLE; Genetic Risk Profile in Longitudinal SLE Cohorts; the Arthritis Research Center Foundation National Data Bank for Rheumatic Disease, the Lupus Foundation of America's Research.forME™Lupus Registry; and the DNA testing company 23andMe's Lupus Research Community. Some studies are closed, and others are still ongoing. I would like to share information about my participation in these observational studies. Don't let the titles scare you; I found participation to be fairly easy—only a few blood draws and urine tests, saliva collection, and completion of several surveys.

---

1 www.clinicaltrials.gov
2 ibid.
3 National Cancer Institute at NIH

My Lupus Research Experiences

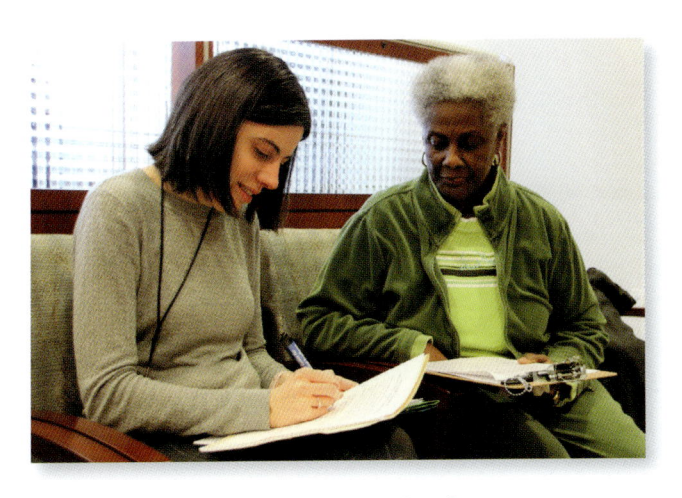

The Fatigue and Lifestyle Physical Activities and SLE Study

Principal investigator: Rosalind Ramsey-Goldman MD, DrPH
Supported by: National Institutes of Health

The study's consent form states, "This study is being done because we would like to see how fatigue, or tiredness, is impacted by physical activity in persons with SLE (systemic lupus erythematosis)." I joined the study on March 19, 2012, and my part in the study lasted less than two weeks.

The study coordinator contacted me during my scheduled lupus clinic visit. We established an appointment in the Clinical Research Unit (CRU) at Northwestern Memorial Hospital to further explain the study and review the consent form. I had to schedule a one-hour visit in the CRU and choose a convenient seven-day period to measure my physical activity by wearing an accelerometer around my waist or wrist.

During my one-hour visit in the CRU, I completed several activities that included review and signing of the consent form; collection of urine; blood draw; assessment of my vital signs by a nurse and my SLE by a physician; completion of two questionnaires; completion of a 20-meter-walk test; and instructions for using and returning the accelerometer. To cover the parking expense, I was given a choice of parking validation or $15.00 in cash.

After wearing the accelerometer for seven days, I returned it to the study coordinator. I also completed a 20-minute telephone interview for the physical activity questionnaire. A check for $50.00 was mailed to me for taking part in the study.

Possible risks that were listed in the consent form included discomfort and minor skin irritation at the section of the waist or wrist where the accelerometer is placed, a bruise or redness at the point where the blood is taken, redness and swelling of the vein, or infection. If some of the questions asked in the surveys made me feel uncomfortable, I could skip them. There was no risk in the walking test. In fact, it was probably a good idea to get the exercise.

By choosing to take part in this study, I gave Dr. Ramsey-Goldman permission to use my personal health information that includes my medical records and information that can identify me—my name, address, phone number, or Social Security number. I also gave permission for all current and previous healthcare providers, including but not limited to the Rehabilitation Institute of Chicago (RIC), Northwestern Medical Faculty Foundation (NMFF), and Northwestern Memorial Hospital (NMH), to give information to the researchers for this study.

The consent form also stated, "Please note that any research information shared with people outside of Northwestern University will not contain your name, address, telephone or Social Security number or any other direct personal identifier unless disclosure of direct identifier is required by law {except that information may be viewed by the study sponsor and its partners or contractors at the Principal Investigator's office}."

My Lupus Research Experiences

Study of Lupus Vascular and Bone Long-Term Endpoints

(SOLVABLE Heart and Bone Study)

Principal Investigator: Rosalind Ramsey-Goldman, MD, DrPH

Supported by: National Institutes of Health, Northwestern Memorial Foundation

The consent form states that the purpose of this study is "to examine the relationship between bone density, or strength of bones, and blood vessel problems in patients with and without lupus. Researchers hope to improve their knowledge regarding common causes of atherosclerosis, an artery disease, and osteoporosis, a disease that gradually weakens bones."

As a participant, I was asked to complete three study visits within a five-year period—April 2012 to April 2017. My first visit lasted about four hours and included four phases. During the first phase in the CRU at Northwestern Memorial Hospital, I was interviewed by a research assistant and examined by a nurse and a doctor. The research assistant asked questions about my medical history, family history, alcohol and tobacco use, and current medications. More questions dealt with my education and work history. I also completed several questionnaires to assess diet, fatigue, overall health status, ability to do daily activities, and my feelings during the past week. The nurse took my height, weight, body measurements, and blood pressure. She also completed a blood draw and collected a urine sample. The doctor did an exam to evaluate my lupus disease status. The first phase lasted one hour, and then I was served lunch.

The second phase of the visit included a bone density test to measure how dense or strong my bones were. In the third phase, I underwent a 45-minute duplex scanning (ultrasound) of my carotid arteries (arteries in my neck) to look for blockages and blood vessel wall thickening. Phase four included an electrocardiogram

(EKG) and imaging of my coronary (heart) arteries and aorta to look for calcium deposits.

After three years of follow-up, a second evaluation was performed. It included all features of the initial visit with the exception of the bone density scan. They also drew additional blood for genetic testing. The third evaluation was performed five years after my initial visit and included another CRU visit and carotid ultrasound scan.

Over the five-year study, I was contacted every six months and asked to report all clinical vascular events (heart attacks, pain, and strokes). By signing the consent form, I gave permission for the principal investigator to review legal papers representing any unfortunate event like hospitalization or death.

As a participant, I gave Dr. Ramsey-Goldman permission to use my personal health information including my medical records and information that can identify me like my name, address, phone number or Social Security number within the Northwestern University (NU) staff and organizations. Records and information disclosed outside of NU would be assigned a unique code number that was to be kept in a locked file. The key to the code was to be destroyed at the end of the research study in April 2017.

Possible risks included low doses of radiation, similar to the exposure received from other routine medical X-rays, and the normal hazards of drawing blood like bruising, inflammation, and infection. Being a participant provided no direct benefit to me except to have some of my test results given to me and my doctor. However, the consent form states that participating in the study "may help to increase scientific knowledge about the relationship between bone density and blood vessel problems in patients with and without lupus."

The study did not interfere with my ongoing medical care with my personal physician. There was no charge for all the tests and

My Lupus Research Experiences

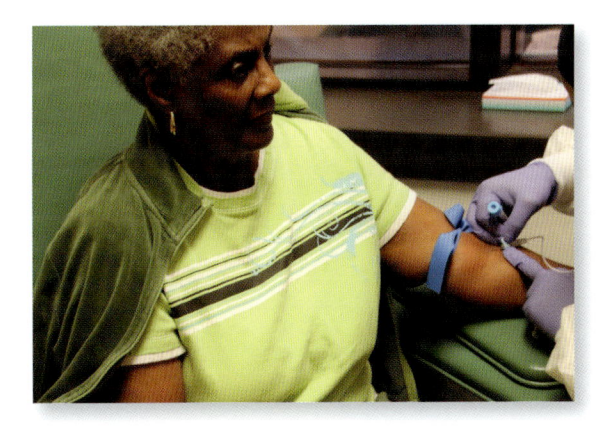

exams. For my participation, I was to receive a $100.00 check within six weeks after each study visit.

SLICC Registry for Atherosclerosis in SLE 9/2012

Principal Investigator: Rosalind Ramsey-Goldman, MD, DrPH
Supported by: Systemic Lupus Erythematosus International Collaborating Clinics (SLICC)

Systemic Lupus Erythematosus International Collaborating Clinics (SLICC) is a group of rheumatologists from twenty-three international centers who have been working since 1991 to carry out lupus research. The researchers report that lupus patients develop atherosclerotic coronary artery disease (thickening of arteries) at a higher rate and earlier age than the general population. The consent form states that the purpose of this study is to develop a registry or database of information on a large number of lupus patients so that researchers may be allowed to "determine the prevalence and nature of early atherosclerotic coronary artery disease in SLE and to identify associated risk factors."

My participation in the study will last for an indefinite period or as long as I wish to be involved. As a participant, I completed a 30-minute interview regarding my physical activity, mental health, age, education, occupation, and family history as it pertains to heart disease. Secondly, the study doctor collected and reviewed my medical records related to lupus, brain and nerve abnormalities, and complications of heart disease.

At my first (baseline) visit, I had blood drawn. The blood was forwarded to the registry's coordinating center for testing of specific risk factors known to be associated with heart disease. Part of the blood was stored for future testing involving genes that may be associated with lupus and with heart disease. After my baseline visit, I am expected to have an annual visit to complete the same activities of interview, review/collection of medical records, and blood draw. Blood draws and record collection/review are forwarded to the coordinating center in Toronto, and I will be informed of any major changes. The study's consent form states that "any blood samples submitted to the coordinating center will be identified by only a study number. The blood samples that are collected will only be used for this research study, and not for any unspecified future projects."

By signing the consent form, I gave SLICC permission to use my personal health information in my medical records and information that can identify me like name, address, phone number, or Social Security number. There is a special note on the consent form that "any research information shared with people outside of Northwestern University will not contain your name, address, telephone or social security number or any other direct personal identifier unless disclosure of the direct identifier is required by law [except that such information may be viewed by the study sponsor and its partners or contractors at the Principal Investigator's office]."

My participation in this study may involve risks such as potential hazards of drawing blood including a bruise at the site of vein puncture, inflammation of the vein, and infection. There is no direct benefit to me; however, the consent form states that "the information collected will be helpful to the study doctor and other researchers in understanding why patients with SLE develop early coronary artery disease, and may provide physicians treating SLE patients with information that will lead to preventive treatment." There is no medical cost to me, nor am I paid for participating.

A Genetic Risk Profile in Longitudinal SLE Cohorts 9/2012

Principal Investigator: Rosalind Ramsey-Goldman, MD, DrPH
Supported by: National Institute of Arthritis and Musculoskeletal and Skin Diseases (NIAMS)/National Institutes of Health (NIH)

The doctors in this study are working with several institutions to find out more about autoimmune disease, its outcome, and why some patients do better than others. The study's consent form states that "there is some evidence that inherited factors (genes) may contribute to the development of autoimmune disease. This study is being done to gain a better understanding of the contribution of inheritance to autoimmune disease occurrence and how inherited properties of the immune system may influence this disease process."

My participation in this study involved a one-hour visit to complete the following: review of my medical records, a 15-minute interview about my health, a blood draw, a urine sample, and a physical exam. I was asked to return once a year for three to eight years to complete identical study visits. The doctors at each participating institution combined information about all study participants from each participating institution. Tests were done at the participating institutions to analyze the antibodies, the inherited factors, and other proteins present. The results of the tests were placed into a database maintained by the National Institutes of Health. My name and other personal identifiers were not added to the database; instead, they were stored under a generic identification number. Only minimal clinical data such as my ethnicity, gender, and lupus diagnosis were included in the database.

The consent form states that possible risks include potential hazards of drawing blood such as bruising at the site of vein puncture, inflammation of the vein, and infection. There is no direct benefit to me, but "the information gained may advance our understanding and treatment of autoimmune diseases such as systemic lupus and related diseases."

There was no cost for exams and tests, and I received $10.00 cash at the end of each visit.

By signing the consent form, I gave researchers permission to use my personal health information in my medical records and information that can identify me like name, address, phone number, or Social Security number. The consent form contains a special note stating that "any research information shared with people outside of Northwestern University will not contain your name, address, telephone or Social Security number or any other direct personal identifier unless disclosure of the direct identifier is required by law [except that such information may be viewed by the Study sponsor and its partners or contractors at the Principal Investigator's office]."

National Data Bank (NDB) for Rheumatic Disease
Arthritis Research Center Foundation, Inc.

On April 2, 2010, I received a letter from Frederick Wolfe, M.D., MACR, the director of the National Data Bank of Rheumatic Diseases (NDB). I'm not sure if I learned about this research from one of my doctors' offices or a magazine. The letter indicated that the NDB was conducting a long-term study of the impact of arthritis and other rheumatic diseases like mine—lupus. The letter stated that, "Through this study we hope to determine the consequences caused by arthritis and other rheumatic diseases and to help guide research into better treatments." I may not receive any direct benefit from this study, but I could be indirectly helping myself "and millions of other people who must live with arthritis and similar conditions."

My Lupus Research Experiences

I was asked to become a participant by signing their consent form and completing a short questionnaire about my medical background and detailed information about medicines. As a participant, I would be expected to give permission to contact my doctors or hospitals for additional information about my care. I would be asked to complete detailed one-hour questionnaires at six-month intervals. The surveys ask questions about arthritis, lupus, my treatments, the effects of the disease on my function, the amount of pain I experience, and the costs that I incur. At first, I completed the questionnaires and returned them through the mail. Now, the questionnaires can be completed online.

Written in the consent form is this statement: "WE CANNOT AND DO NOT GUARANTEE OR PROMISE THAT YOU WILL RECEIVE ANY BENEFITS FROM THIS STUDY, but your participation will help increase knowledge of and interest in arthritis and other rheumatic diseases." NDB claims no risk or cost is involved, and no payment will be provided.

By signing the consent form, I authorized the use and disclosure of my health information that is collected in connection with this research study. However, my information will not be disclosed to anyone in any way that would reveal my identity, except to federal and regulatory agencies as required. The consent form also states that "any data that may be published in scientific journals will not reveal the identity of the subjects."

This is a long-term study with no fixed number of months or years, and I am free to withdraw my consent and discontinue my participation at any time.

Lupus Foundation of America's Research.forME Registry

I receive emails from the Lupus Foundation of America (LFA) on a regular basis. In April of 2017, my eyes were drawn to an article titled "What Does Research Mean to You?" The article included a description of an interesting idea that would allow the voice of lupus patients to be heard throughout the whole research process. LFA's Research.forME Registry, an online registry for the lupus community, is a place for people living with lupus or those taking care of a loved one with lupus to provide information about their life with the disease. This program provides a space to share experiences, to help design research questions, and to receive information about findings or studies that matter to the patient.

I joined the registry in June of 2017 and completed an online survey with screening questions that helped determine my eligibility. The second step was to review and affirm my consent to participate. Finally, I needed to complete a more detailed 45-minute web-based survey. At the beginning of this survey, I was given the opportunity to choose one of four options for the level of involvement. The first option involved being a part of the lupus registry that collects information about your experience with lupus and receiving information about studies that specifically match your needs. The second option was being part of a lupus research interest group that receives news about studies that are relevant to you. The third one required being a volunteer for PARTNERS, a patient-powered research network that brings together families affected by childhood rheumatic diseases such as lupus, several patient advocacy organizations, and clinicians who work to improve health care and advance lupus research. Checking the fourth option of "no thanks" indicated not having an interest in any of these options at that time.

I chose the first option—to share my lupus experiences. Therefore, periodically, I complete short surveys about living with lupus. I also receive information about topics and research studies of interest to me. Recently, I received this message from the program:

"We are reaching out to tell you about a Lupus Foundation of America survey. As part of a grant with the United States Centers for Disease Control and Prevention (CDC PULSE Grant No. 6

My Lupus Research Experiences

NU58 DP006139-02), we are doing a survey to understand the self-management needs and habits of people who have lupus. Information from the survey will be used to develop a new web-based program to help people with lupus manage their condition and improve their well being.

After successful completion of the survey, you will be invited to enter a raffle for one of ten $25 Target gift cards, one $250 gift card, or one $500 gift card."

Being a member of the registry provides an opportunity for my voice to be heard in lupus research. The information that I share could help shape lupus research studies and help researchers and patients understand lupus better. I will also receive information about lupus research studies.

For more information, contact the registry coordinator online at registrycoordinator@lupus.org.

The Lupus Research Community
23andMe Lupus Study
Founder: Pfizer Inc.

"Currently, the cause of lupus is unknown, but previous research suggests that there is a strong genetic component involved. The 23andMe web-based platform enables a large group of individuals with lupus to come together to provide valuable data for research. This research data includes genetic information (using DNA from saliva) and information about each participant's unique experiences with the disease (using responses from online surveys). Conducting research using this data may help improve diagnosis and find better treatments" (lupus-help@23andme.com). Understanding the role of genetics in lupus could be a crucial step towards prevention, accurate diagnosis, treatment, and eventually, a cure.

Fighting Lupus Battles

In 2015, I discovered that the DNA testing company 23andMe was recruiting up to 5,000 lupus patients to participate in their research project with Pfizer, one of the world's largest pharmaceutical companies. This study is focused on two main areas: genetic factors that may contribute to the cause and severity of lupus and how genes might influence different responses to medications or other treatments (23andme.com).

I enrolled in the study and signed a consent form that allowed 23andMe to collect, store, and complete research on my genetic data, medical records, and survey answers. My contribution mainly involved the initial saliva collection and completion of surveys about how lupus affects my daily activities and my general physical and emotional health. If I agree to more genetic research, I might need to contribute annual blood draws and complete semi-annual surveys. I provided a sample of my saliva to be stored in the 23andMe laboratory for genetic analysis. I own my genetic data and can withdraw from the study at any time; however, my saliva sample, once submitted to and analyzed by 23andMe, is processed in an irreversible manner and cannot be returned to me.

I agreed to allow 23andMe and Examination Management Services, Inc. (EMSI) to contact my physician and request my medical records, including my lab results, appointment summaries, and diagnoses. EMSI is an independent third-party service provider that specializes in contacting health providers to obtain medical records. I was told that the information from my medical records would be securely transferred to 23andMe and used by EMSI only for that purpose. It was spelled out in the Authorization to Release Confidential Medical Information that my protected health information would be used by 23andMe and Pfizer and would be stored in the 23andMe secure database. My health information would be shared and exchanged with Pfizer as de-identified information—that is, my data will be stripped of

My Lupus Research Experiences

any identifying components such as my name, address, email address, user ID, or password. My authorization remains in force as long as 23andMe maintains my health information or considers it to be useful for scientific, research, educational, statistical or public health purposes.

Over the course of one year, I completed seven short online surveys. The surveys included questions about my diagnosis, treatment, symptoms, medications, and family history. I received Amazon gift certificates of $5.00 immediately after I completed each of five surveys and $25.00 after I completed the last survey in November of 2016.

23andMe plans to compare my genetic data, medical records, and survey answers with other research participants. To increase the chance that meaningful scientific discoveries about lupus are made, 23andMe may share my de-identified data with qualified research partners, such as Pfizer, global researchers, and global scientists. If 23andMe shares my genetic or self-reported data with a qualified research partner, this action cannot be undone, and my data will not be returned to 23andMe.

23andMe cites the two risks revolving around storage of genetic information and survey answers. The company guarantees that it has built all their systems to maximize protection of individual data and made it extremely difficult for employees or external parties to link identifying information to DNA results and survey responses. However, if there is a security breach, my data could be leaked. Also, I may learn information about myself that I had not anticipated. For example, I might learn surprising facts related to my ancestry like being related to a family member in a way that is different from the way I thought.

This project provides an opportunity to take a direct role in research that may benefit me and other individuals with lupus. Other benefits include being able to participate in web-based research

Fighting Lupus Battles

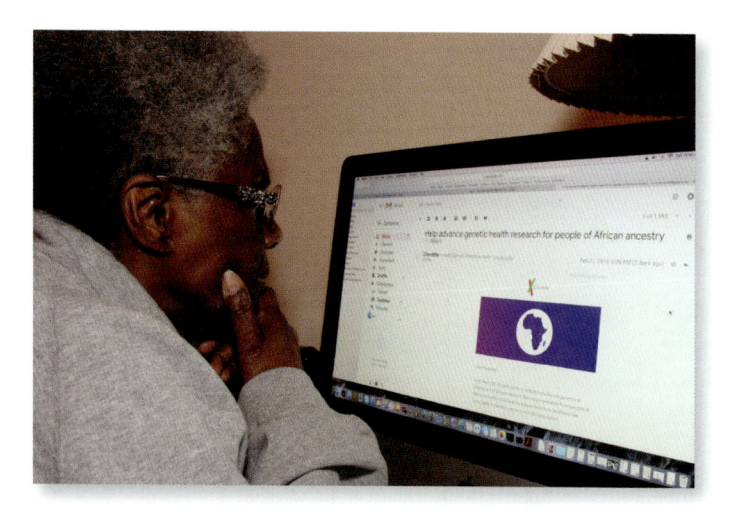

from the comfort of my own home, being kept informed of the discovery process as research advances, and having the option to learn more about my genetic ancestry. The testing for new customers was free, and participants received compensation up to $50 total for completing the surveys.

In December of 2017, I received this notice: "Thank you for partnering with 23andMe in our efforts to better understand the underlying genetic factors that contribute to lupus. Your contributions will go a long way. The study is now officially closed and we are beginning our data analysis."

***

Though my participation was limited to these five observational studies, I feel good about my contribution to lupus research. At first, I had reservations about privacy and confidentiality, especially when I was asked to provide my Social Security number. However, I decided that the potential benefits outweighed my reservations. I look forward to the discoveries that may benefit the lupus community. Hopefully, we can move swiftly toward discoveries that will lead us to the cause, prevention, early diagnosis, safer and more effective treatment options, and a cure.

Development of Patient-Reported Outcomes Tools

Meenakshi Jolly, MD, MS

Do you want to tell your doctor how lupus and its treatments affect your daily life in an effective and efficient manner? Dr. Meenakshi Jolly recommends using LupusPRO (Patient Reported Outcomes), Body Image in Lupus Screen (BILS), and Lupus Impact Tracker (LIT), surveys developed for just this purpose.

Dr. Jolly is a professor in the Department of Medicine and the Department of Behavioral Sciences, associate director in the Rheumatology Fellowship Program, and director of the lupus clinic at the Rush University Medical Center in Chicago. She is actively engaged in research on patient-reported health outcomes and psychosocial health in lupus patients. Dr. Jolly has worked on developing tools to measure and communicate the effects of lupus or its treatment on the daily lives of lupus patients.

LUPUS MAY AFFECT your physical, emotional, personal, social, professional, and economic health. The patient may be the only one who really knows how lupus uniquely affects his or her daily life. Yet, frequently, lupus patients find it difficult to communicate with their doctors. Some reasons for the difficulty may include having limited time during visits, forgetting to mention items you meant to discuss, being uncomfortable and not knowing the best way to communicate some issues, and feeling that the issue might not be a priority for the doctor. Doctors usually spend their time talking about symptoms, examining the patient, reviewing and discussing laboratory tests and other investigations (e.g. X-rays), developing a management plan, discussing and monitoring medications, their side effects, and much more. Dr. Jolly states that she learns about lupus patients and their concerns by working closely with them and explaining expected benefits and harms of proposed treatments in friendly and relatable language. She further states that using rigorous scientific research methods like LupusPRO, Body Image in Lupus Screen, and Lupus Impact Tracker have resulted in her ability to learn more about various ways in which lupus or its treatment impacts their daily lives.

LupusPRO has 43 questions. It was derived from male and female lupus patients from diverse racial and ethnic groups in the United States and uses gender-neutral language. It was designed specially for patients with lupus. LupusPRO was designed to measure:

- lupus symptoms/flares
- concerns about pregnancy
- brain fog
- side effects of lupus medicines
- satisfaction with care
- effects of disease on your career, desires, and goals
- coping
- social support

LupusPRO also includes the Body Image in Lupus Screen (BILS) that assesses pain, vitality, sleep, physical and emotional health, and planning. The Lupus Impact Tracker has only ten questions and provides an easy and fast way for lupus patients and their doctors to communicate and track your disease. (http://www.lupuspro.com)

According to Dr. Jolly, these research methods help to improve communication between patient and doctor, especially when time during a routine doctor visit is limited. This enables doctors to give patients the appropriate care they deserve. It also fosters

Development of Patient-Reported Outcomes Tools

shared decision-making, personalized care, and patient-doctor relationship. Patients who are better educated about their condition and feel that their physician understands and attends to their unique health issues is more likely to be satisfied with their care, more engaged in their own care, and more likely to follow their management plan.

Dr. Jolly reports that these tools have been studied widely—not only in the US but also in many other countries and in various languages. She says that they have been published in various scientific journals and presented in numerous national and international conferences. She verifies that the tools have been tested and found to function well among patients of various countries, languages, and cultures. Dr. Jolly recommends that patients use either of these surveys to follow your disease progression and treatment, as well as to communicate your concerns to your doctors. Ask your doctor about how you can access this tool to improve the quality of your care.

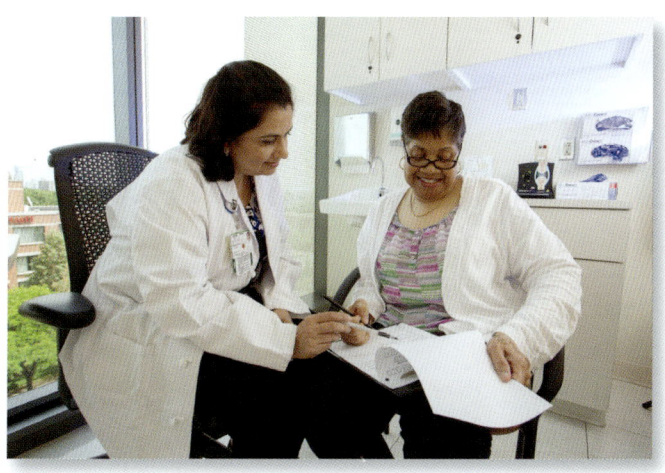

Dr. Jolly, left

Bench-to-Bedside Model
Kichul Ko, MD

Dr. Ko is an assistant professor of medicine in the Section of Rheumatology at the University of Chicago Gwen Knapp Center for Lupus and Immunology Research.

LUPUS KIDNEY DISEASE, called lupus nephritis, is one of the most serious complications of lupus. It can lead to proteins being spilled in the urine and eventual kidney failure. A patient with lupus nephritis can have increased risk of blood clots and heart disease as well as infection. Despite advancement in diagnosis and therapy, lupus nephritis patients may still not do well as up to half of patients with severe lupus nephritis can end up in dialysis. Dialysis is a medical treatment to replace the functions of kidneys when these organs fail. Just as kidneys do, dialysis can filter blood and maintain stable levels of important chemicals in the blood such as potassium and sodium. These patients need aggressive medications, but there are also large concerns about potential side effects from them.

At the University of Chicago's Gwen Knapp Center for Lupus and Immunology Research directed by Marcus Clark, MD, we have been trying to study lupus nephritis using the "bench-to-bedside" model—from laboratory research to clinical studies and trials. By using this model, we hope to discover what is actually going on in the patients' kidneys that are being affected by lupus and develop potential targets for therapy. Traditionally, lupus nephritis has been classified based on changes that occur on kidney structures called *glomeruli* where blood filtration occurs. Although healthy glomeruli are vital to normal kidney function, the majority of the kidney is made up of another structure called tubulointerstitial (TI) space, through which filtered blood travels and important cells reside.

A few years ago, our group led by Christine Hsieh, MD, observed that lupus nephritis patients with moderate-to-severe inflammation occurring in the TI space did worse than those with minimal-to-mild inflammation. On the other hand, when the patients were divided based on the changes in the glomeruli (the traditional way to classify lupus nephritis), no difference was seen. So the next logical question that arose was, *what is actually happening in the TI space in the kidneys of patients with lupus nephritis?*

This question was then taken to the "bench"—the laboratory. Scientists from our group such as Anthony Chang, MD, and Andrew Kinloch, PhD, used kidney biopsy samples of lupus patients to show differences. There were groups of immune cells in the TI space of lupus kidneys that acted differently from those in the rest of the body. The immune cells in the kidney formed their own self-propagating system and produced local autoantibodies that were different from systemic autoantibodies such as double-stranded DNA antibodies (systemic autoimmunity). So, we questioned whether our current medications actually target both the systemic autoimmunity and this separate, distinctive immune system in the TI space in the kidney

One type of the local autoantibodies we found in the TI space is called an anti-vimentin antibody. These were found in higher numbers in lupus patients with nephritis compared to those without, and definitely higher in those with severe TI inflammation. We are currently studying whether these antibodies can be used in diagnosis, prognosis, or treatment targets in lupus nephritis.

Studying human kidney tissues can be very challenging for a number of reasons. First, the biopsy samples are only snapshots.

Fighting Lupus Battles

We cannot view the cellular interactions in real-time the way researchers can in mice. Also, the cells are very close to each other, making it difficult for scientists to tell them apart. Moreover, scarring can occur in lupus nephritis, and this can interfere with the way we see these cells. To combat this problem, our group, led by Vladimir Liarski, MD, has developed a computer program that can convert analog microscope images into digital images. This allows us to figure out the shapes of cells in kidneys, the number of specific cells we are interested in, and how they interact based on the distance between the cells. Since everything is done in an objective automated manner, there is less room for bias and human errors.

Using this automated technique, our group, led by Kichul Ko, MD, in collaboration with a pharmaceutical company, demonstrated that a molecule called Bcl-2 was abnormally elevated in many immune cells in the TI space in the kidneys of our lupus nephritis patients. We then hypothesized whether Bcl-2 could be a potential target for treatment. By studying mice that had lupus similar to humans, we were able to show that by lowering the levels of Bcl-2, we were able to prevent these mice from developing lupus nephritis and therefore improve their survival.

Currently, at the University of Chicago, several other projects are ongoing, and they range anywhere from laboratory research (bench) to clinical studies and trials (bedside). In addition to efforts from several scientists and physicians in our group, the most help comes from our patients and their willingness to participate in research so that we can continue to move forward in trying to find better ways to diagnose and treat lupus.

For more information, visit us at *lupus.uchicago.edu*.

The Activity in Lupus to Energize and Renew (ALTER) Study

Rosalind Ramsey-Goldman, MD, DrPH

Dr. Ramsey-Goldman is the Solovy Arthritis Research Society Professor of Medicine at Northwestern University's Feinberg School of Medicine.

What is the problem and what is known about it so far?

Systemic lupus erythematosus (SLE, lupus) is a systemic auto-immune disease characterized by pronounced inflammation that affects up to 1.5 million persons in the US. One of the main problems for those who suffer from lupus is chronic, debilitating fatigue that significantly decreases quality of life, increases risk of work disability, and is associated with significant healthcare costs. An urgent, unmet need in the management of patients with SLE is to find ways to reduce fatigue. This need was highlighted in the recent report summarizing the Lupus Patient-Focused Drug Development (PFDD) meeting held in September 2017.

Non-pharmacological interventions (treatments that don't use medication) including physical activity were reported to have potential to be effective in decreasing fatigue in persons with SLE. For example, one study documented the quantity and perceptions of physical activity in 50 persons with SLE, in which only 14 out of the 50 (28%) reported that they met the US government's public health goal of at least 150 minutes per week of moderate to vigorous intensity activity. Although 92% of the study's participants believed that physical activity was beneficial for SLE and that they could be more physically active, more than 78% believed that

SLE impeded their ability to exercise. The persons with SLE in this study expressed fears about getting injured during exercise, but they thought physical activity would be good if it were managed appropriately for those with a chronic illness. We also need more data on sleep, depression, anxiety, and pain—conditions that also contribute to fatigue.

Why did the researchers do this particular study?

We determined that a research study is needed to improve understanding of the relationship between fatigue and key aspects of physical activity (how often, how long, how easy or hard). This type of study would be a step toward developing better and more efficient intervention programs including physical activity for persons with SLE. In order to accurately measure the amount of the patients' physical activity, we used an accelerometer (a wearable instrument like a pedometer that measures steps). To fully understand some of the factors contributing to fatigue in persons with SLE, we also needed to measure sleep problems, depression, anxiety, and pain. For that part of the study, we used the Patient-Reported Outcomes Measurement Information System (PROMIS) tools.

Who was studied?

129 persons with SLE were studied.

How was the study done?

After obtaining informed consent, 129 persons with SLE wore an accelerometer on their waist for one week. This tool measured the amount and the intensity of their physical activity during the week. The participants also answered questions about fatigue, sleep, pain, and physical function. To assess depression and anxiety over the last week, patients responded to questions about how they were feeling.

The ALTER Study

What did the researchers find?
We were able to measure the amount and intensity of physical activity in 129 patients wearing the accelerometer for one week. The amount of physical activity was related to the amount of fatigue reported by the patient; Lower amounts of physical activity were related to more fatigue. We also discovered that the majority of the patients did not meet the US guidelines for physical activity in adults. The scores for the patient-reported outcomes were worse for the persons with lupus compared to the general US population. More intense physical activity was associated with less pain, less fatigue, and better physical function.

What were the limitations of the study?
This was a small study. In this small study, we could not show a relationship between physical activity and sleep, depression, or anxiety. The measurements were done only once and may not reflect the person's usual activity, i.e. during the study a participant may have been on holiday or off of work for other reasons. The participants may have changed their physical activity because they were wearing the accelerometers. The patient-reported outcomes only reflect the week prior to the assessment and may not reflect their quality of life concerns over time.

What are the implications of the study?
We are able to measure physical activity and patient-reported outcomes in lupus. These tools can be used for intervention studies aimed toward measuring fatigue and the impact of physical activity on fatigue. We have designed a clinical trial to test several educational and behavioral strategies to decrease fatigue in lupus. The trial is called the Lupus Intervention Fatigue Trial (LIFT). You can find it on clinicaltrials.gov and the registration number is NCT02653287. Recruitment will start in the second half of 2018.

This study was supported by NIH/NIAMS grant R21 AR059989.

Fighting Lupus Battles

References

Ahn GE, Chmiel JS, Dunlop DD, Helenowski IB, Semanik PA, Song J, Ainsworth B, Chang RW, Ramsey-Goldman R. "Self-reported and objectively measured physical activity in adults with systemic lupus erythematosus." *Arthritis Care & Research* 67, no. 5 (2015): 701-707.

Mahieu MA, Ahn GE, Chmiel JS, Dunlop DD, Helenowski IB, Semanik P, Song J, Yount S, Chang RW, Ramsey-Goldman R. "Fatigue, patient reported outcomes, and objective measurement of physical activity in systemic lupus erythematosus." *Lupus* 25, no. 11 (2016) :1190-1199

Ahn GE, Ramsey-Goldman R. "Fatigue in systemic lupus erythematosus." *International Journal of Clinical Rheumatology* 7, no. 2 (2012): 217-227.

Mahieu M, Yount S, Ramsey-Goldman R. "Patient-Reported Outcomes in Systemic Lupus Erythematosus." *Rheumatic Diseases Clinics of North America* 42, no 2 (2016): 253-263.

Lupus Research Alliance Delivering Research Breakthroughs to Transform Lupus Treatment

Teodora P. Staeva, PhD

Dr. Staeva is the research director of the Lupus Research Alliance.

NEW TREATMENT OPTIONS for lupus are urgently needed. Only four drugs are commonly used to treat lupus, and most have some serious side effects. The Lupus Research Alliance (LRA) is committed to changing this landscape by funding the most promising research and facilitating clinical translation to improve treatments while driving toward a cure.

Over the past nearly 20 years, the LRA has invested more than $200 million in lupus research programs with nearly 500 studies that advance our understanding of lupus, help develop new treatments, and bring us closer to the cure. Indeed, LRA-funded research has contributed to the identification or further validation of at least 15 different disease pathways in lupus that are currently being targeted by over a dozen different drugs.

Key Research Successes in Lupus Treatment

As a result of a research approach grounded in innovative and foundational science with an eye to the clinic, LRA-supported scientists have produced pivotal discoveries in the genetics, immunology, and organ involvement of lupus. For instance, the LRA funded the initial research studies that eventually led to the development of Benlysta, the first new lupus treatment in more than 60 years and the only one developed specifically for lupus. Another example of success: the LRA commissioned a comprehensive analysis of existing drugs for their potential use as lupus treatments and, based on those findings, recommended that Janssen Pharmaceuticals test their psoriasis drug Stelara as a treatment for lupus. Results so far have been promising, and testing of Stelara for lupus continues in a phase 3 trial. The organization has also supported numerous basic research projects that identified and validated the critical role of the type I interferon pathway in lupus, which is currently targeted by different therapeutic approaches in clinical development.

2018 Brings Breakthrough Discoveries

In 2018 alone, scientists funded by the LRA have made many important findings. For instance, at the National Institute of Arthritis and Musculoskeletal and Skin Diseases (NIAMS), Dr. Mariana Kaplan and colleagues found that abnormal immune system cells are damaging patients' arteries. Published in the journal *JCI Insight*, these findings provide more evidence for research of experimental drugs that target these cells to potentially protect people with lupus from heart attacks and strokes.

A new study by LRA-funded researcher Dr. Matthew Weirauch of the Cincinnati Children's Hospital Medical Center in Ohio and colleagues might explain how a common virus that causes mononucleosis also boosts the risk for lupus. The virus may be turning on human genes that promote the illness. The scientists, including co-authors Dr. John Harley and Dr. Leah Kottyan of the Cincinnati Children's Hospital Medical Center, are now looking at several compounds that may block the virus' effects.

Another study co-funded by the LRA has produced a significant discovery about the role of bacteria and points to the potential for a vaccine or treatment that might prevent an autoimmune attack by suppressing specific bacteria. Led by Dr. Martin Kriegel at Yale University, the study was published in the prestigious journal *Science*. As reported by Yale University, Dr. Kriegel's team discovered that the bacteria *Enterococcus gallinarium*, normally found in

LRA Delivering Research Breakthroughs

the small intestine, could travel to other organs like the liver and trigger an autoimmune attack. When testing tissue from people with lupus, they found that both an antibiotic and a vaccine could stop the bacteria's growth in the liver, thereby preventing the autoimmune response. Additionally, they were able to target *E. gallinarum* specifically, avoiding effects on the other bacteria in the intestine.

Also, with support from a LRA Novel Research Grant, Dr. Robert Anthony of Massachusetts General Hospital successfully turned autoimmune antibodies that attack a person's own cells into antibodies that instead reduce tissue damage. Published in the journal *Cell*, this discovery could lead to a new, effective treatment of lupus and other autoimmune diseases.

As a recipient of the LRA Distinguished Innovator Award, Dr. Zhijian (James) Chen at the University of Texas Southwestern Medical Center identified a mechanism that stimulates the immune system. This discovery could lead to novel treatments for infections, lupus and other autoimmune diseases, and cancer. Published in *Science*, his discovery concerning an enzyme called cGAS uncovered an essential process that alerts the immune system to viruses by sensing the presence of "foreign DNA within cells." Dr. Chen was able to confirm his hypothesis that this pathway malfunctions in lupus, causing the immune system to mistakenly attack its own DNA. That breakthrough reveals a strong potential target for therapies to treat or prevent lupus and other autoimmune diseases by blocking the enzyme cGAS.

A study with important implications for lupus classification and clinical trials was also published in 2018 in *Annals of the Rheumatic Diseases*. Led by Dr. David Pisetsky of Duke University School of Medicine and conducted as part of the LRA's Lupus Industry Council, the study showed that not all individuals who have been diagnosed with lupus remain positive for antinuclear antibodies (ANA), despite the long-held scientific belief to the contrary.

Importantly, this study also reveals that whether a person with long-standing lupus tests ANA-positive or negative can vary widely depending on the particular ANA test being used. These findings have implications for identifying patients eligible for clinical trials and raise important questions about the natural history of disease progression in individuals with established lupus.

LRA Testing Potential Treatments Through Trial Network

In addition to providing grants to scientists around the world, the LRA formed the Lupus Clinical Investigators Network (LuCIN) to speed the identification, development, and testing of new lupus treatments. LuCIN is made up of leading lupus experts at top research centers throughout the US and Canada. LuCIN funds a wide range of clinical trials from exploring a new app to make reporting symptoms to an individual's lupus doctor easier, to testing investigational compounds as potential lupus treatments.

Visit LupusTrials.org to find out about ongoing lupus studies to consider joining. In addition, learn more about our funded research and its latest discoveries through our main website, LupusResearch.org.

About the Lupus Research Alliance (LRA)

The LRA aims to transform treatment while advancing toward a cure by funding the most innovative lupus research in the world. The organization's stringent peer review process fosters diverse scientific talent who are driving discovery toward better diagnostics, improved treatments, and ultimately a cure for lupus. Because the LRA's Board of Directors funds all administrative and fundraising costs, 100% of all donations goes to support lupus research programs.

The Lupus Research Community

Scott Hadly

Scott Hadly is a managing editor at 23andMe, Inc.

We at 23andMe, Inc. understand that the study of underlying genetics of lupus could lead to better diagnostics and more effective treatments with fewer side effects. With 23andMe, Inc. having the largest community of customers who've consented to participate in research, we offer a unique opportunity for this kind of genetic research. In 2015, 23andMe, Inc., in collaboration with Pfizer Pharmacy, Inc., launched recruitment efforts for the research community.

The research is focused on understanding the genetic factors associated with developing lupus and the differences in the progression and severity of the disease. We want to better understand the role of genetics and how patients respond to different treatments. We would also like to apply this understanding to drug targeting and development efforts.

This research collaboration with Pfizer included a recruitment phase, a data collection phase, and then a study phase. We are still completing the work on the later stages of this study. An institutional review board (IRB) oversees the research. The IRB is an independent panel of experts who ensure the research meets ethical and legal guidelines. This study also included input from a group of external advisors from lupus research advocacy groups and medical researchers who specialize in lupus research.

Fighting Lupus Battles

Participants had to meet certain eligibility requirements, including having a lupus diagnosis, an ability to access the Internet, and consent for their medical records to be accessed by the study researchers. Some participants were recruited from among existing 23andMe customers. Some were recruited using social media.

We rapidly completed the recruitment phase in December 2017 with 5,000 participants. We are still working on the data collection and study phases, which include a one-year longitudinal study. Our plan is to publish our findings at a future date and share those findings with participants.

Research.forME™ Lupus Registry
The Lupus Foundation of America

The Lupus Foundation of America (LFA) is a nonprofit organization devoted to solving the mystery of lupus. We aim to improve the quality of life for all people affected by lupus through research, education, and advocacy. Within our research program, we lead and fund original ideas and studies, including our Research.forME initiative that was launched in April 2017. Research.forME is a suite of programs and services that encourages people with lupus to participate in every step of the research process. The steps range from taking part in a focus group discussion about a study that has not been developed yet to helping develop culturally relevant study recruitment materials. Currently, Research.forME includes a patient registry that connects people with opportunities of interest to them, a lupus research interest group, and educational resources on clinical trials.

The Research.forME Registry is part of an observational, quantitative study. This means we are using numbers and statistics to talk about trends in people with lupus, including symptoms, diagnosis time, or treatment. An institutional review board (IRB) approves the study. The IRB ensures participants and their personal information are protected and that data is collected and handled ethically. Individuals who would like to enroll in the registry will be given an informed consent form to review and agree to before joining. This outlines what their participation means, the benefits and risks of taking part, and who they can contact with questions. There are no known risks, and while there are no immediate personal benefits, the study might lead to future benefits for people with lupus.

Fighting Lupus Battles

The Lupus Registry is a place to store detailed information about people diagnosed with lupus. People of all ages with lupus and their legal caregivers are able to join. Participants can choose to share information about their lupus experience through a survey. The survey takes about 35 minutes to complete and covers topics from healthcare access to how lupus affects people's daily lives. After a participant enrolls, LFA will send occasional emails with opportunities to participate in research studies that match the information they provided. We envision participants being able to log on and see clinical trials or surveys that match their profile. This will make research more personalized and interesting to the lupus community.

Other disease areas, like cystic fibrosis or Alzheimer's, have similar databases for matching patients with clinical trials. These databases have been successful in getting more patients involved in research, which we hope will happen with lupus. People with lupus can be involved at all stages of research, which will help make participation easy to understand and more tailored to what patients want. The registry gives patients a voice that will guide the direction of clinical research in lupus and future treatments. Findings from the registry have not been published to date, but we plan to conduct ongoing analysis of our findings.

People who have not yet been diagnosed but still want to be involved can sign up for the Lupus Research Interest Group. This is similar to the Lupus Registry, but it is not a formal study. Participants answer more general questions about themselves and their symptoms. They still receive news on research studies based on their responses. Members of both the Lupus Research Interest Group and the Lupus Registry can also volunteer for a patient-powered research network called PARTNERS (Patients, Advocates and Rheumatology Teams Network for Research and Service), which brings together families, patient advocacy organi-

Research.forME Lupus Registry

zations like LFA, and doctors to improve healthcare and research for children affected by rheumatic diseases such as lupus.

The Research.forME Lupus Registry and Lupus Research Interest Group provide valuable information about lupus and the people it affects. Community members, researchers, drug companies, and policy makers are only some of the groups that will benefit from this research. LFA wants to hear directly from patients and their caregivers. This gives us the chance to better understand and tackle lupus from all directions and get more people with lupus interested in research. Research will pave the way to a life free of this cruel disease.

To learn more and enroll in the Research.forME Lupus Registry, visit resources.lupus.org/registry.

Part III
Summary

In 2015, the National Institute of Arthritis and Musculoskeletal and Skin Diseases (NIAMS) prepared the Action Plan for Lupus Research that included this statement: "Lupus is difficult to diagnose; may cause attacks on any organ in the body including skin, joints, heart, lungs, kidneys, and brain; may require some treatments that can have many side effects; is chronic—forever; can be disabling, even fatal, and has no cure... YET."[1]

The American College of Rheumatology echoes NIAMS' optimistic outlook on the future of lupus treatments, saying, "there is much reason for hope. Improvements in treatment have greatly improved these patients' quality of life and increased their lifespan."[2]

There have been many benefits from participation in lupus research. A report from NIAMS shows that sixty years ago, about fifty percent of those with lupus were likely to have a significantly compromised quality of life and could even die within five years. NIAMS also states that the treatments for lupus were of limited effectiveness; therapies were associated with significant and often debilitating side effects; diagnosis of lupus was more difficult; and "sophisticated tools of molecular medicine were not yet available." There is evidence that living with lupus today has improved drastically over what it was like yesterday. NIAMS reports that people

---

[1] https://www.niams.nih.gov/about/working-groups/lupus-federal/action-plan

[2] https://www.rheumatology.org/I-Am-A/Patient-Caregiver/Diseases-Conditions/Lupus

who are diagnosed with lupus today have hope for a significantly increased life span and improved quality of life compared with those diagnosed thirty years ago. Researchers have solved some of the mysteries, yet there are still many questions about lupus. Here are two major questions.

What causes lupus?

No one seems to know. NIAMS says that "research suggests that genes play an important role, but genes alone do not determine who gets lupus. It is likely that many factors trigger the disease."[3] The NIH/NIAMS pamphlet *Living With Lupus* reports, "The environment, sunlight, stress, and certain medicines may trigger symptoms in some people. Other people who have similar genetic backgrounds may not get signs or symptoms of the disease. Researchers are trying to find out why."

Who gets lupus?

Scientists report that anyone can be diagnosed with lupus. The NIAMS Action Plan notes that "recent independent surveys have suggested a prevalence as high as 1.5 million in the USA. Women with the disease outnumber men nine to one. Lupus often strikes women in their early working and childbearing years, interfering with the ability to work, have or raise a family, or in some cases, even care for themselves."[4] It is also documented that lupus is more prevalent in African Americans, Asian Americans, Latino/Latina Americans, and Native Americans than Caucasian populations. Why? That's another mystery.

I believe that participation in clinical studies is a valuable tool to help answer these and other questions about lupus. The National Institutes of Health explains that "clinical studies are designed to add to medical knowledge related to the treatment, diagnosis,

---

[3] https://www.niams.nih.gov/health-topics/lupus
[4] https://www.niams.nih.gov/about/working-groups/lupus-federal/action-plan

Summary

and prevention of diseases or conditions."[5] We need more clinical research so that we'll be able to increase knowledge about lupus, to get an earlier diagnosis, to develop better treatment plans, and to discover how to prevent and eventually cure lupus.

The National Institutes of Health states that "groundbreaking medical advances will only happen through clinical research participation."[6]

We need more research projects, more participants, more scientists, and more sponsors. We all can be involved in helping us move toward prevention, more efficient diagnostic process, better treatment plans, and a cure for lupus. However, Kenneth Getz notes in his book, *The Gift of Participation,* that most people are reluctant to participate in research:

> "Only 2% of the American population gets involved in clinical research each year. Among people who suffer from severe, chronic illnesses, only 6% participate. As a result, an increasing number of clinical trials are delayed because too few people are willing—or even knew they had the opportunity—to get involved.
>
> "Most people appreciate the value of clinical research and say they are likely to participate in a study. Yet no more than a third of those who identify and qualify for a clinical trial choose to enroll."

Low participation levels in clinical research studies continues to be a problem. The CISCRP has discovered that "upwards of 80% of clinical research studies struggle with the need to find more participants."[7] We need to do better. The National Institutes of

---

5   https://www.clinicaltrials.gov/ct2/about-studies/learn
6   https://www.nih.gov/sites/default/files/health-info/clinical-trials/why-nih-clinical-research-matters.ppt
7   www.nih.gov/sites/default/files/health-info/clinical-trials/why-nih-clinical-research-matters.ppt

Fighting Lupus Battles

Health warns that a lack of participants in research can seriously impact whether a study is successful.[8]

There is evidence that though we still don't have a cure or know the definite causes, living with lupus today has improved drastically over what it was like yesterday. The NIAMS notes that "the past two decades of research have yielded a wealth of new information and growth in improving our understanding of lupus. Today, thanks to advances brought about by research, 97 percent of lupus patients are living five years after diagnosis, and 90 percent continue to survive after ten years."[9] Let's move to the next level and find ways to prevent and cure lupus.

After reading this section, I hope that more people will gain insight into the need for and importance of lupus research, have a better understanding of the lupus research process, become aware of the need for more volunteers in lupus research, and feel more comfortable volunteering to participate in lupus research. According to NIH, patient involvement helps researchers to uncover better ways to prevent, diagnose, treat, and understand human disease. What can you do to help solve the mysteries of lupus? You could begin by asking your doctors about ways you might contribute to lupus research. Learn more about lupus research at ClinicalTrials.gov. and other resources listed in this book.

---

8   ibid.
9   NIAMS Action Plan for Lupus Research, www.niams.nih.gov/about/working-groups/lupus-federal/action-plan

References and Resources

Organizations

23andMe, Inc.
www.23andme.com

American College of Rheumatology (ACR)
www.rheumatology.org
2200 Lake Boulevard NE
Atlanta, GA 30319
Phone: 404-633-3777
Fax: 404-633-1870

Mission: "To empower rheumatology professionals to excel in their specialty. We are a professional membership organization committed to improving the care of patients with rheumatic disease and advancing the rheumatology subspecialty."

Centers for Disease Control and Prevention (CDC)
www.cdc.gov
Phone: 800-CDC-INFO (800-232-4636)

Mission: "CDC increases the health security of our nation. As the nation's health protection agency, CDC saves lives and protects people from health threats. To accomplish our mission, CDC conducts critical science and provides health information that protects our nation against expensive and dangerous health threats, and responds when these arise."

Fighting Lupus Battles

Center for Information and Study on Clinical Research Participation (CISCRP)

www.ciscrp.org
One Liberty Square, Suite 510
Boston, MA 02109
Phone: 877-MED-HERO (877-633-4376)

Mission: "A non-profit organization founded in 2003 and dedicated to educating the public and patients and to engaging these critical stakeholders as partners in the clinical research process, CISCRP provides a variety of award-winning and internationally recognized educational resources, programs and services including print and digital materials; media outreach and awareness campaigns, live educational events; study volunteer appreciation programs; patient advisory boards and custom research assessing patient health journeys and study volunteer experiences; and plain language clinical trial results summaries."

Lupus Foundation of America, Inc.

www.lupus.org
2121 K Street NW, Suite 200
Washington, DC 20037
Phone: 202-349-1155 or 800-558-0121
Fax: 202-349-1156

"Our mission is to improve the quality of life for all people affected by lupus through programs of research, education, support and advocacy."

References and Resources

Lupus Research Alliance
www.lupusresearch.org
276 Madison Avenue, 10th Floor
New York, NY 10016
Phone: 212-218-2840 or 800-867-1743

Mission: "The Lupus Research Alliance is the world's leading private funder of lupus research. Established in 2016—from the merger of the Alliance for Lupus Research, the Lupus Research Institute, and the S.L.E. Foundation—the Lupus Research Alliance was created to improve treatments for lupus while advancing toward a cure. This effort includes raising funds and advocating on behalf of the lupus community in the public policy arena."

Lupus Society of Illinois (LSI)
www.lupusil.org
411 S. Wells Street, Suite 503
Chicago, IL 60607
Phone: 312-542-0002 or 800-258-7872;

Mission: "LSI promotes lupus awareness and complements the work of health care professionals by providing personalized resources for the lupus community while supporting research."

National Cancer Institute (NCI) at the National Institutes of Health (NIH)
www.cancer.gov
9609 Medical Center Drive
Bethesda, MD 20892-9760
Phone: 800-4-CANCER (800-422-6237)

Mission: "NCI leads, conducts, and supports cancer research across the nation to advance scientific knowledge and help all people live longer, healthier lives."

Fighting Lupus Battles

FORWARD—The National Data Bank for Rheumatic Diseases
www.ndb.org
1035 N Emporia, Suite 288
Wichita, KS 67214

National Institute on Arthritis and Musculoskeletal and Skin Diseases (NIAMS) at the NIH

www.niams.nih.gov
1 AMS Circle
Bethesda, MD 20892
Phone: 301-495-4484 or 877-22-NIAMS (877-226-4267)

Mission: "The mission of the National Institute of Arthritis and Musculoskeletal and Skin Diseases, as part of the U.S. Department of Health and Human Services, National Institutes of Health (NIH), is to support research into the causes, treatment, and prevention of arthritis and musculoskeletal and skin diseases; the training of basic and clinical scientists to carry out this research; and the dissemination of information on research progress in these diseases."

National Institutes of Health

www.nih.gov
9000 Rockville Pike
Bethesda, Maryland 20892
Phone: 301-496-4000

Mission: "The National Institutes of Health (NIH), a part of the U.S. Department of Health and Human Services, is the nation's medical research agency—making important discoveries that improve health and save lives."

References and Resources

National Institutes of Health Clinical Center and ResearchMatch Patient Recruitment
clinicalcenter.nih.gov/recruit/ResearchMatch.html
Phone: 800-411-1222
TTY 866-411-1010

"The NIH Clinical Center has joined ResearchMatch, an online, national clinical research registry that "matches" people who want to participate in clinical studies with researchers who are seeking volunteers. ResearchMatch is a free and secure web-based service that helps connect volunteers to clinical studies taking place at the NIH Clinical Center in Bethesda, Maryland, and at other major academic institutions across the country. All institutions are part of the NIH Clinical and Translational Science Awards program." (clinicalcenter.nih.gov)

Research.forME Lupus Registry
resources.lupus.org/registry

US Department of Health and Human Services
Office of Women's Health
200 Independence Avenue, SW
Washington, DC 20201
Phone: 800-994-9662
womenshealth.gov

Online Resources

Clinical Trials and You: The Basics
www.clinicaltrials.gov

"The ClinicalTrials.gov website provides current information about clinical research studies to patients, their families and caregivers, health care professionals, and the public. Each study record includes a summary of the study protocol, including the purpose, recruitment status, and eligibility criteria. Study locations and specific contact information are listed to assist with enrollment. (See How to Read a Study Record to learn more about the information found in a study record.) Information on ClinicalTrials.gov is provided and updated by the sponsor or principal investigator of the clinical study. Clinicaltrials.gov is a free service of the National Institutes of Health (NIH) and is maintained by the National Library of Medicine (NLM)"

MedlinePlus
www.medlineplus.gov

Mission: "MedlinePlus is the National Institutes of Health's Web site for patients and their families and friends. Produced by the National Library of Medicine, the world's largest medical library, it brings you information about diseases, conditions, and wellness issues in language you can understand. MedlinePlus offers reliable, up-to-date health information, anytime, anywhere, for free."

NIAMS Action Plan for Lupus Research
Published December 22, 2015
www.niams.nih.gov/sites/default/files/files/action_plan_lupus.pdf

NIAMS/NIH Booklet: "Living with Lupus"
https://www.niams.nih.gov/sites/default/files/catalog/files/LivingWithLupus_English.pdf

NIH PowerPoint: "Why NIH Clinical Research Matters"
www.nih.gov/sites/default/files/health-info/clinical-trials/why-nih-clinical-research-matters.ppt

The Lupus Foundation of America's Expert Series: Lupus Brain Fog by George Tsokos, MD
https://www.lupus.org/resources/the-expert-series-lupus-brain-fog

Publications

Kenneth Getz, *The Gift of Participation: A Guide to Making Informed Decisions About Volunteering for a Clinical Trial* (Bar Harbor, Maine: Jerian Publishing, 2014).